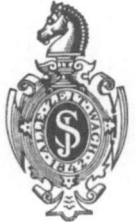

Drug-Induced Injury to the Digestive System

M. Guslandi M.D.

Gastroenterology Unit,
S. Raffaele Hospital and
Dept. of Biomedical Sciences,
University of Milan, Italy

P. C. Braga M.D.

Department of Pharmacology,
Chemotherapy and Toxicology,
School of Medicine,
University of Milan, Italy

Springer-Verlag
Berlin Heidelberg New York London Paris
Tokyo Hong Kong Barcelona Budapest

With 13 Figures

ISBN-13: 978-88-470-2222-5   e-ISBN-13: 978-88-470-2220-1
DOI: 10.1007/978-88-470-2220-1

© Springer-Verlag Berlin Heidelberg 1993
Softcover reprint of hardcover 1st edition 1993

Typesetting: Mitterweger GmbH, Plankstadt, Germany
65/3145-5 4 3 2 1 0 – Printed on acid-free paper

Foreword

Every day millions of people in the world take drugs to obtain pain relief, decrease a high temperature, overcome an infection, heal a tissue injury, restore some altered body function, or fight cancer. Drugs are precious tools to acquire and maintain health. Their proper use is one of the most challenging issues in medical science (and the art of medical practice). Unfortunately, the main therapeutic effect of every drug is accompanied by side effects, some of which represent adverse, undesirable reactions.

Since drugs are often introduced into the body by the oral route it is no wonder that the digestive system is by far the most frequent target of untoward drug-induced effects. Much has been written on this topic, but the information is scattered throughout the medical literature, sometimes in toxicological journals that physicians seldom have the opportunity to read. On the other hand, the books which in the past have addressed the issue are now long outdated owing to the rapid and unrelenting evolution of medical therapy.

We believe that for the benefit of all the physicians who every day face the problem of possible, presumed, or established drug-induced adverse effects on the digestive system a new, updated volume is overdue. Thus, with the help of a group of distinguished authors, each a recognized expert in his field, we have assembled this volume, which we hope will be helpful to anyone (physicians, researchers, pharmacologists) involved in the medical profession.

MARIO GUSLANDI
PIER CARLO BRAGA

Contents

List of Contributors

BERTOLISSI, E.; Division of Gastroenterology and Digestive Endoscopy, Regional Cancer Center, Aviano, Italy

BORTOLUZZI, F.; Division of Gastroenterology and Digestive Endoscopy, Regional Cancer Center, Aviano, Italy

BRAGA, P. C.; Department of Pharmacology, School of Medicine, University of Milan, Milan, Italy

BJARNASON, I.; Departments of Clinical Biochemistry and Medicine, King's College School of Medicine and Dentistry, London SE59PJ, U.K.

CANNIZZARO, R.; Division of Gastroenterology and Digestive Endoscopy, Regional Cancer Center, Aviano, Italy

CASPARY, W.F.; Abteilung für Gastroenterologie, Zentrum der Inneren Medizin, Universitätsklinikum, Frankfurt/Main, BRD

CHAUDHURI, T. K.; Veterans Affairs Medical Center, Hampton, Virginia 23667, USA

FERGUSON, R.; Wirral Hospital, Upton, Wirral, Merseyside, U.K.

FINK, S.; Veterans Affairs Medical Center, Hampton, Virginia 23667, U.S.A.

FORNASARIG, M.; Division of Gastroenterology and Digestive Endoscopy, Regional Cancer Center, Aviano, Italy

GUSLANDI, M.; Gastroenterology Unit, S. Raffaele Hospital and Department of Biomedical Sciences, University of Milan, Milan, Italy

KÖLBEL, B. C.; Abteilung für Gastroenterologie, Medizinische Klinik, Universitätsklinikum, Essen, BRD

LAMOULIATTE, H.; Service des Maladies de l'Appareil digestif, Hôpital Saint-André, Bordeaux 33075, France

LANGMAN, M. J. S.; Department of Medicine, Queen Elizabeth Hospital, Birmingham B15 2TH, U.K.

LARREY, D.; Service d'Hépato-gastroentérologie, Hôpital Saint-Eloi, Montpellier, France

LEMBCKE, B.; Abteilung für Gastroenterologie, Zentrum der Inneren Medizin, Universitätsklinikum, Frankfurt/Main, BRD

MACPHERSON, A.; Departments of Clinical Biochemistry and Medicine, King's College School of Medicine and Dentistry, London SE59PJ, U.K.

MÜLLER-LISSNER, S.; Medizinische Klinik, Klinikum Innenstadt, Ludwig-Maximilians-Universität, München, Germany

QUINITON, A.; Service des Maladies de l'Appareil digestif, Hôpital Saint-André, Bordeaux 33075, France

SANDOR, Z.; Chemical Pathology Research Division, Department of Pathology, Brigham and Women's Hospital and Harvard Medical School, Boston, MA, USA

SINGER, M. V.; Medizinische Klinik für Gastroenterologie, Fakultät für Klinische Medizin, Universität Heidelberg, Mannheim, BRD

SOZZI, M.; Division of Gastroenterology and Digestive Endoscopy, Regional Cancer Center, Aviano, Italy

SZABO, S.; Chemical Pathology Research Division, Department of Pathology, Brigham and Women's Hospital and Harvard Medical School, Boston, MA, USA

VALENTINI, M.; Division of Gastroenterology and Digestive Endoscopy, Regional Cancer Center, Aviano, Italy

WEHRMANN, T.; Abteilung für Gastroenterologie, Zentrum der Inneren Medizin, Universitätsklinikum, Frankfurt/Main, BRD

WILSON, S.; Veterans Affairs Medical Center, Hampton, Virginia 23667, USA

ZERBIB, F.; Service des Maladies de l'Appareil digestif, Hôpital Saint-André, Bordeaux 33075, France

Drugs and the Mouth

R. FERGUSON

Wirral Hospital, Upton, Wirral, Merseyside, U.K.

Drugs may damage the mouth in a variety of ways. Some of the reactions are predictable, such as those of cytotoxics by immunosuppression or direct cytotoxic effect and those of certain antibiotics by encouraging candidal infections, while others are unpredictable, for example, hypersensitivity reactions (antibiotics, barbiturates).

1 Diseases of the Oral Mucosa

1.1 Glossitis

Drugs causing chronic gastrointestinal blood loss, for example, nonsteroidal anti-inflammatory drugs (NSAIDs), may ultimately cause iron deficiency and hence glossitis. Folate deficiency may similarly cause a red, sore, depappilated and smooth tongue. Folate deficiency may be drug induced by an uncertain mechanism, such as anticonvulsant and oral contraceptive agents, or by acting as inhibitors of dihydrofolate reductase, a key enzyme in the metabolism of folate. Such inhibitors include methotrexate, trimethoprim, triamterene and pyrimethamine. Antifungal agents such as amphotericin, nystatin, miconazole, keto- conazole and griseofulvin may cause median rhomboid glossitis, a red depappilated area in the centre of the tongue.

1.2 Glossodynia

The sensation of a burning tongue may be drug induced, but it is more commonly an expression either of an anxiety or a deficiency state. It can be associated with candidiasis or xerostomia (see below). Long-term griseofulvin therapy [1] is a common cause, often being associated with a black appearance of the tongue. Captopril and perhaps to a lesser extent the other angiotensin-converting enzyme inhibitors enalapril, lisi- nopril, fosinopril, perindopril, quinapril and ramipril may cause glosso- dynia [2,13].

1.3 Oral Ulceration

All cytotoxic agents may cause mouth ulceration, usually as a result of immunosuppression. Other drugs causing oral ulceration unrelated to immunosuppression are penicillamine, emepromium bromide, isoprena- line tablets, chlorhexidine mouthwashes and proguanil. Oral ulceration may follow the use of local irritants if kept in the mouth for a prolonged period of time. Such drugs include aspirin, potassium preparations and pancreatin [3,1].

1.4 Erythema Multiformae

In this condition and in the more severe form, the Stevens-Johnson syn- drome, there are extensive painful areas and ulcers of the cheek, tongue and palatal mucosa. A haemorrhagic gingivitis is common. Although a variety of drugs may cause this, the commonest are sulphonamides, bar- biturates and penicillin.

1.5 Stomatitis Medicamentosa

This condition characterized by erythema of the tongue and mucosal membranes in the mouth is often caused by broad-spectrum antibiotic therapy, presumably as a result of alteration of the flora of the mouth, and it may be associated with candidiasis (see below). All NSAIDs may cause this, as may penicillamine and a variety of chemotherapeutic agents. A stomatitis secondary to a hypersensitivity reaction has been reported following phenolphthalein, phenacitin, phenazone, amidopyrine, phenindione, indomethacin, antibiotics and barbiturates [9].

2 Xerostomia

This is a common complaint caused by drugs with anticholinergic or sympathomimetic effects; tricyclic antidepressants are also a common cause. The drugs causing dry mouth in long-term use are shown in Table 1. Xerostomia is a common side effect of cancer chemotherapy [10] and such patients are particularly sensitive to infection from normal oral flora and the development of oral ulceration. Candidiasis is also common.

Table 1. Drugs causing dry mouth in long-term use

Drugs with anticholinergic effects
Atropin, ipratropium, hyoscine and analogues
Orphenadrine, benzhexol and related anti-parkinsonian agents
Tricyclic antidepressants
Antihistamines
Major tranquilizers, particularly phenothiazines
Anti-emetics
Some antihypertensive agents, especially ganglionblockers and clonidine

Drugs with sympathomimetic actions
"Cold cures" containing ephedrine, etc.
Bronchodilators
Decongestants
Appetite suppressants
Amphetamines

Diuretics
Diazide
Amiloride
Frusemide

3 Pigmented Mucosal Lesions

Although these occur for a variety of reasons, for example, racial characteristics, smoking, heavy-metal poisoning, Albright's syndrome, haemachromatosis, neurofibromatosis and incontientia pigmenti, they may be caused by phenathiazine [13].

4 Ageusia

Total absence of taste caused by drugs is rare. Dysgeusia is more common. Single cases of ageusia have been reported after treatment with the antifungal agents griseofulvin and terbinafin, the antihypertensive captopril, cefacotril, oxyfedrine, penicillamine and thiouracil. The cause of ageusia by these agents is unknown.

5 Dysgeusia

Although many drugs may alter the sensation of taste, the reason for this is unknown. A list of such agents is shown in Table 2.

6 Candidiasis

Half the population have species of Candida as oral commensals [14]. Whether these commensals cause candidiasis is unknown, but antibiotic therapy and drugs leading to xerostomia predispose to oral candidiasis. Of the four clinical varieties of candidiasis, only denture wearers contract chronic atrophic candidiasis, manifesting itself as a diffuse erythema of the palate under the denture, with occasional white patches and angular cheilitis. Acute pseudomembraneous candidiasis (thrush) is a disease of infancy and debilitated adults and is not usually drug related. This condition is characterized by symptomless white patches or exudates which, when rubbed, leave an erythematous mucosa. By contrast, acute atrophic candidiasis is a painful condition characterized by a smooth, red tongue and cheilitis and is caused by antibiotic therapy. Any antibiotic may be a causative agent. Cytotoxic agents and other drugs which cause immunosuppression, for example, steroids, may be associated with this type of candidiasis.

7 Diseases of the Gingiva

7.1 Gingival Bleeding

Although gingival bleeding is common and generally caused by gingivitis, gingival haemorrhage may be secondary to thrombocytopenia. Thrombocytopenia may be caused by many drugs, including cytotoxic agents, or a hypersensitivity reaction to almost any drug. Gingival bleeding may also be caused by anticoagulant therapy (e.g. warfarin, phenindione) but tends to occur only when the dose of such drugs is above the therapeutic range.

Table 2. Drugs affecting taste

Classification	Drugs
Agents for dental hygiene	Sodium lauryl sulfate (toothpaste)
Amoebicides and antihelmintics	Metronidazole, Miridazole
Anaesthetics, local	Benzocaine, procaine hydrochloride and other, cocaine hydrochloride, tetracaine hydrochloride
Anticholesteremic	Chlofibrate
Anticoagulants	Phenindione
Antihistamines	Chlorpheniramine maleate
Antimicrobal agents	Amphotericin B, ampicillin, cefamandole, griseofulvin, ethambutol hydrochloride, lincomycin, sulphasalazine, streptomycin, tetracyclines, tyrothricin
Antiproliferative, including immunosuppressive agents	Doxorubicin and methotrexate, azathioprine, carmustine, vincristine sulphate
Antirheumatic, analgesic, antipyretic, anti-inflammatory agents	Allopurinol, cholchicine, gold, levamisole, D-penicillamine, phenylbutazone, 5-thiopyridoxine
Antiseptics	Hexetidine
Antithyroid agents	Carbimazole, methimazole, methylthiouracil, propylthiouracil, thiouracil
Diuretics and antihypertensive agents	Captopril, diazoxide, ethacrynic acid
Hypoglycaemic drugs	Glipizide, phenformin and derivatives
Muscle relaxants and drugs for treatment of Parkinson's disease	Baclofen, chlormezanone, levodopa
Opiates	Codeine, hydromorphone hydrochloride, morphine
Psychopharmacologic, including anti-epileptic drugs	Carbamazepine, lithium carbonate, phenytoin, psilocybin, trifluoperazine
Vasodilators	Oxyfedrine, bemifylline hydrochloride
Others	Industrial chemicals, including insecticides, germine monoacetate, idoxuridine, iron sorbitex, vitamin D

7.2 Gingival Hyperplasia

Phenytoin is the commonest drug to cause this condition. Characteristically the interdental papillae are first involved, later the rest of the gingiva. The gingival sites involved are usually the buccal and labial; palatal, lingual and edentulous sites are rarely involved. The gingiva involved is firm and pale with a stippled appearance. These appearances may take years to develop. Early lesions may be soft and red. Such changes are most pronounced in the first year of treatment and may resolve if the drug is withdrawn. Neither the patient's age, sex, phenytoin dosage, nor the phenytoin serum concentration is an important determinant of the severity or incidence of hyperplasia. There is, however, a clear relationship to poor oral hygiene. Other drugs, including the calcium antagonists nifedipine, diltiazem and verapamil, may cause gingival hyperplasia. Cyclosporin may also cause this condition in children. The mechanism of gingival overgrowth due to drug may involve an action between the drug or a metabolite and the gingival fibroblast enhanced by inflammation. This in part may be genetically determined [7]. Other hypotheses include a drug-induced increase in fibroblast receptors to epidermal growth factor [12], inactivation of collagenases [7], inhibition of calcium iron uptake by fibroblasts and the subsequent increase in the proliferation rate [6] and, in respect to phenytoin, a decrease in cellular folate [4]. As folate is vital for collagenase activator proteins, a deficiency of it results in a lack of saturable collagenase for connective tissue catabolism, resulting in gingival overgrowth.

8 Dental Caries and Tooth Disease

Prolonged intake of drugs with a high sucrose content may predispose to dental caries. A further cause is prolonged drug-induced immunosuppresion. Chemotherapeutic agents, by causing immunosuppression and xerostomia, are a potent cause of dental caries. Tetracycline administration to young children can cause permanent yellow staining of the fixed dentition. Prolonged overdosage of vitamin D may cause disturbance of dental enamel leading to bacterial invasion of the pulp and loss of the tooth.

References

1. Bramble MG, Record CO (1978) Drug induced gastrointestinal disease. Drugs 15: 451–463
2. British National Formulary, 24, 87–89
3. Brown RD, Bolas G (1973) Isoprenoline ulceration of the tongue. A case report. Br Dental J 134: 336–337
4. Drew H, Vogel R, Molofsky W, Baker H, Frank O (1987) Effect of folate on phenytoin hyperplasia. J Clin Periodontol 14: 350–356
5. Ferguson R (1987) Diseases of the mouth. In: Diseases of the gut and pancreas, 1st ed Blackwell, Oxford, 79–89
6. Fuji A, Kobayashi S (1990) Nifedipine inhibits calcium uptake of Nifedipine sensitive gingival fibroblasts. J Dent Res 67: 332

7. Hassell TM (1982) Evidence for production of an inactive collagenase by fibro-blasts from phenytoin-enlarged human gingiva. J Oral Pathol 11: 310–317
8. Hassell TM, Gilbert GM (1983) Phenytoin sensitivity of fibroblasts as the basis for susceptibility to gingival enlargement. Am J Pathol 112: 218–223
9. Kay LW (1972) General and local ulceration problems. In: Drugs and dentistry, 2nd Ed Wright, Bristol, 263–264
10. Leggott PJ (1990) Oral complications in the paediatric population and oral com-plication of cancer therapy. NCI Monogr 9: 129–132
11. Meyler's side effects of drugs (1988) 11th ed, 568
12. Modeer TM, Anderson G (1990) Regulation of epidermal growth factor receptor metabolism in gingival fibroblasts by phenytoin in vitro. J Oral Pathol Med 19:188–191
13. Scully C, Porter SR Diseases of the oral mucosa (1990) Med Int 3154–3161
14. Shiffman SS (1983) Taste and smell in disease. N Engl J Med 308: 1275–1279, 1337–1343

Drug-Induced Esophagitis

A. QUINTON, F. ZERBIB, and H. LAMOULIATTE

Service des Maladies de l'Appareil digestif, Hôpital Saint-André, Bordeaux, France

Although drugs have been administered since antiquity, esophageal injuries caused directly by prolonged contact with tablets or capsules have only recently been recognized. The first case of esophageal ulceration following oral potassium therapy was described in 1970 [37]. Since then, many cases have been reported in the literature, and more than 50 drugs have been involved. Drug-induced esophagitis is observed only rarely, occurring in less than 1% of cases [18]. A survey of a population of 700,000 over a 4-year period in Sweden reported an incidence of 3,9 cases per 100,000 population per year [11]. Nevertheless, the incidence may be underestimated. Many cases are not reported since the course is usually favorable, and many more are probably unrecognized or attributed to other esophageal diseases, in spite of characteristic clinical features and endoscopic findings [7, 21]. Esophagoscopy is necessary for diagnosis, control of the complete mucosal healing, and detection of distant complications.

1 Drugs Involved

Three drugs have been associated with 75 % of the cases of esophageal injury: emepronium bromide, antibiotics, and potassium chloride.

Emepronium bromide is an anticholinergic quaternary ammonium compound, used to relieve urinary frequency and for incontinence in the United Kingdom, Germany, Switzerland, and Scandinavia, but not approved for use in the United States or France. Emepronium bromide tablets can cause ulceration of both mouth and esophagus. More than 60 cases of esophageal injury have been reported since Habeshaw and Bennett described the first case [24].

Antibiotics have been associated with more than 50 % of esophageal injury cases, doxycylin representing 80 % of these cases [5, 27]. Despite replacement of doxycline capsules by tablets, these lesions remain a complication of this therapy. The list of antibiotics involved in esophageal injuries is reported in Table 1.

Potassium chloride is dispensed as non coated, coated, or slow-release tablets. Although esophageal ulcers and stenosis have been reported with non coated tablets [40], the coated slow-release tablets are usually implicated, mainly in elderly patients with cardiomegaly [5, 27].

Drug-induced esophagitis has been reported with many other drugs: ferrous sulfate, steroidal and nonsteroidal anti-inflammatory drugs (first aspirin and piroxicam), quinidine, alprenolol, associated with aspirin and dextropropoxyphene, and pinaverium bromide are the most frequently implicated drugs (see Table 1). Recently, zidovudine-related esophageal ulcerations have been reported in three HIV-infected patients [17].

2 Incidence

The age of patients with drug-induced esophagitis reflects the population group most likely to receive the commonly prescribed drugs. Injuries from tetracyclines and emepronium bromide occur in young patients (mean age of cases being 30 and 34 years, respectively), whereas potassium chloride-induced esophagitis is more frequently observed in elderly patients with cardiac disorders (mean age 51 years) [18]. There is an increased use of aspirin and nonsteroidal anti-inflammatory drugs (NSAIDs) for the treatment of arthritis in middle-aged patients [19]. The frequency of drug-induced esophagitis is the same among male and female patients. The high frequency of urinary symptoms in this group explains the predominance of females in patients with emepronium bromide-induced esophageal injuries [21].

3 Clinical Presentation and Outcome

3.1 Symptoms

Symptoms are usually acute and closely follow the ingestion of the causative agent, in most cases during the first month of treatment. Symp-

Table 1. Drug induced esophagitis: drugs involved

Antibiotics

Tetracyclines
  Doxycycline[b]
  Methylenecycline
  Minocycline[a]
  Oxytetracycline
  Tetracycline hydrochloride[a]
Penicillins
  Amoxycillin
  Apocillin
  Cloxacillin
  Phenoxymethyl penicillin
  Pivmecillinam

Others
  Clindamycin
  Cotrimoxazole
  Erythromycin
  Lincomycin
  Spyramycin
  Sulfamethoxypyridazine
  Tinidazole

Cardiovascular drugs

Alprenolol[a]
Captopril
Digoxin
Mexiletine
Naftidrofuryl

Propranolol
Quinidine[a]
Tetranitrate
Warfarin

Nonsteroidal anti-inflammatory drugs

Aspirin[a]
Ibuprofen
Indomethacin

Meclofenamate
Phenylbutazone
Piroxicam[a]

Miscellaneous

Allyl sulfide
Ascorbic acid
Benzalconium chloride
Carbachol
Clinitest[a]
Chlorazepate dipotassium
Cromolyn sodium
Dexamethasone-aspirin
Dextropropoxyphene-aspirin[a]
Dextropropoxyphene-paracetamol
D-Penicillamine
Emepronium bromide[b]
Estramustin phosphate
Ferrous sulfate[a]
Fluorouracil
Mequitazin

Oxybutinin
Papain
Percogesic
Phenacetin-aspirin-caffeine
Phenobarbital
Phenyltoxolamine-paracetamol
Phenytoin
Pinaverium bromide[a]
Potassium chloride[b]
Prednisolone
13-*cis* Retinoic acid
Theophylline
Thiamin-calcium-cystin
Thiazinamium
Zidovudine

---

[a] 5–20 cases reported.
[b] > 20 cases reported.
Other drugs, fewer than 5 cases reported.

toms may develop a few days after withdrawal of the drug, but the reason is not clear. A firm protective eschar resulting from the coagulation necrosis of the esophageal mucosa may delay the development of symptoms until it sloughs off [34]. Emepronium bromide induced lesions often occur later than lesions induced by tetracyclines. In most cases, the drugs are swallowed with only a small amount of fluid and often shortly before going to bed or resting in supine position [5, 34].

The pattern of complaints is characteristic: the first symptom is frequently the sensation of a foreign object located retrosternally. Then retrosternal pain, heartburn, odynophagia, and dysphagia are the most common manifestations [31]. Hematemesis and melena may also result from drug-induced esophageal damage [14, 41].

3.2 Diagnosis

Confronted with a suggestive history, flexible fiberoptic endoscopy is very sensitive in establishing the diagnosis of drug-induced esophagitis, revealing one or several superficial erosions or ulcers and in some cases pill remnants retained within the esophagus [27, 34, 37]. The lesions are frequently irregular and maplike, less frequently round or oval, and occasionally encompass the entire circumference of the esophagus [18]. Small ulcers are often seen, ranging from pinpoint size to 60 mm, usually produced by antibiotics, emepronium bromide, or NSAIDs. These tiny flat erosions become further evident with a Lugol's solution vital staining [35]. Patients injured by potassium chloride or quinidine tablets are more likely to have deep ulcers and smooth or ulcerated strictures. Deep ulcers usually have edges that bleed easily and are surrounded by profuse white exsudate [27]. However, brown and blue-green overlying exsudates have been described respectively in ferrous sulfate and doxycycline-induced ulcers [1, 32]. The most common site of drug-induced esophageal injury is the mid esophagus ("suspended ulceration"), at the level of the aortic arch, an area characterized by external compression, the skeletal to smooth muscle transition, and by the physiologic reduction of the amplitude of the esophageal peristaltic waves. Lesions are found in the lower third of the esophagus in about 20 % of cases [19, 27]. The mucosa below and above the lesion is typically normal, but a hiatal hernia or a localized stricture might contribute to pill retention [20].

Esophageal biopsies show nonspecific acute inflammation, ulceration and edema, without fungi or viral (herpes, cytomegalovirus) inclusion bodies [27]. Nevertheless, one case of methylenecycline-induced ulcer with mycosis superinfection has been reported [36]. Single-contrast radiography shows changed only in severe cases where there are deep ulcers or stricture [19]; double-contrast studies are reported to be more sensitive and useful, detecting subtle mucosal abnormalities and superficial ulcers [8]. However, in many cases the barium esophago-gram is normal, and endoscopy is much more sensitive than radiography in establishing a diagnosis of drug-induced esophagitis [3].

3.3 Outcome and Complications

Most tetracyclines and emepronium bromide-induced injuries have a favorable outcome [16]. After withdrawal of the offending medication and symptomatic treatment, patients usually improve within a week. Esophagoscopy reveals complete mucosal healing after 3–6 weeks of treatment [5, 7, 27]. Only a single fatal outcome has been reported with doxycycline in a patient affected with an Ehlers-Danlos syndrome [40].

The most common complications are esophageal strictures, essen-tially induced by potassium chloride and quinidine tablets, occurring most frequently in elderly subjects [6, 30]. Pill-induced esophageal strictures are more common than previously reported; they may be confused with those secondary to gastroesophageal reflux. The diagnosis is suggested by a history of drug ingestion, the location of the stricture in the mid esophagus, and a normal 24-h esophageal pH monitoring. In most cases, dilatation of the stricture is sufficient to relieve dysphagia. Esophageal resection with colon interposition is exceptionally required when dilata-tions are not successful [6]. Less common complications include bleed-ing [29, 41, 44], and esophageal perforation sometimes leading to death and usually occurring with potassium bromide or NSAIDs [7, 29, 31].

4 Pathophysiology

Both delayed transit of the pill through the esophagus and direct injury of the mucosa are implicated in the incidence and severity of drug-induced esophagitis.

4.1 Delayed Transit Time of Pill Within Esophagus

"Dry" swallowing and supine position are the two principal risk factors for the occurrence of a delayed transit time. Evans and Roberts [20] have shown that barium sulphate tablets, similar in size to aspirin, can remain in the esophagus longer than 5 min, and up to 90 min in patients who swallow the tablets with a small amount of water (15 ml) and then lay flat. Esophageal retention occurred in 52 % (36/69) of normal sub-jects and in 72 % (21/29) of subjects with a radiologically abnormal eso-phagus. Many other studies confirm the poor clearance of tablets from the esophagus when ingested without enough fluids and/or in a supine position [2, 12, 26]. In addition, sleep is known to reduce salivation, swallowing and esophageal peristaltism, and the sleeping patient is unaware of any discomfort [16, 33]. The influence of size and shape of commonly used medication has also been studied. Hey et al. [26] showed that large oval tablets and capsules pass through the esophagus faster than large round tablets when taken with 25 ml water, but the difference was not apparent when 100 ml was taken; however, small tablets had a significantly faster transit time than large tablets, irrespective of the amount of water taken. Furthermore, doxycycline tablets proved much less apt to lodge in the esophagus than hard gelatin capsules, which become sticky when moist and have a tendency to adhere to the mucosa and dissolve locally [10]. Likewise, hydrophilic swelling agent incorporated into 100- and 200-mg emepronium bromide tablets may be responsible for excessive adherence of such tablets [3, 28, 38].

Other factors are also implicated in impairment of esophageal transit time. Delay in passage of the tablets is more likely to occur in patients with motility disorders [5], hiatus hernia and gastroesophageal reflux with or without stricture [20], and in patients with extrinsic compression from cardiomegaly with an enlarged left atrium (particularly those receiving potassium chloride tablets) [13, 19, 37]. Additionally, emepronium bromide is not only an irritative medication but by its anticholinergic action may induce gastroesophageal reflux, thereby further contributing to damage [19].

4.2 Mechanism of Direct Injury

A potential caustic acidic effect is incriminated in drugs with low pH (<3) which can be dissolved in the esophageal lumen, not only tetracyclines but also aspirin, ascorbic acid, and ferrous sulfate [7, 16, 27]. However, acidity alone cannot account for the ulcerogenic effect and other mechanisms may explain injuries induced by pills such als clindamycin, emepronium bromide, and potassium chloride which do not produce acidic solutions. Doxycycline, when held within the esophagus wall, accumulates in the basal layer of squamous epithelial cells and causes hemolysis [22]. In a recent study, Bailey et al. [4] showed the influence of the dissolution rate of drugs. Frequently, multiple ulcers may be found in the same patient, due to a non uniform dispersion of capsule contents after disintegration [15]. NSAID-induced esophageal injuries may be related to direct toxicity caused by inhibition of mucosal prostaglandin synthesis and disruption of the mucosal barrier, especially when associated with gastroesophageal reflux [7, 25, 42].

Rentention of slow-release potassium chloride tablets within the esophagus leads to local accumulation of ionized potassium, which may cause intramucosal vascular spasms, infarction, and consequent ulceration, hemorrhage, perforation, and sometimes stricture. The same mechanism is involved in the potassium-induced small bowel lesions [5, 7].

Accidental ingestion of Clinitest tablets, as they dissolve, causes direct thermal injury of the mucosa [9].

5 Prevention and Treatment

5.1 Prevention

Patients should be advised to take drugs with at least 100 ml fluid, in the upright position, and well before going to bed. Slow-release potassium chloride tablets should be replaced by liquid preparations, and doxycycline-coated tablets are to be preferred since they are less frequently associated with esophageal ulcerations than non-coated forms [16]. These forms should be preferred in elderly and/or bedridden patients, especially if they have an abnormal esophagus or a cardiomegaly [43].

5.2 Treatment

Withdrawal of the offending medication is the first step and, if not feasible, replacement by either a parenteral or liquid form. Most reported cases have been treated for 2–3 weeks with antacids, H_2 blockers [5, 31] or a sucralfate suspension, which has the advantage of binding to the ulcer [23, 39]. In addition, if the esophageal lesions are associated with gastroesophageal reflux, alginic acid, and metoclopramide can be prescribed [5], and patients with complete odynophagia may benefit from use of a topical anesthetic agent [7].

References

1. Abbarah TH, Fredell JE, Ellenz GB (1976) Ulceration by oral ferrous sulfate. J Am Med Assoc 286: 2319–2320
2. Applegate GR, Malmud LS, Rock E et al (1980) "It's a hard pill to swallow" or "don't take it lying down". Gastroenterology 78: 1132
3. Barrison IG, Trewby PN, Kane SP (1980) Esophageal ulceration due to emepronium bromide. Endoscopy 12: 197–199
4. Bailey RT, Bonavina L, Nwakama PE, De Meester TR, Cheng C (1990) Influence of dissolution rate and pH of oral medications on drug-induced esophageal injury. DICP, The Annals of Pharmacotherapy 24: 571–574
5. Becouarn Y, Lamouliatte H, Quinton A (1983) Lésions aiguës de l'œsophage d'origine médicamenteuse. Gastroenterol Clin Biol 7: 868–876
6. Bonavina L, De Meester TR, MacChesney L et al (1987) Drug-induced esophageal strictures. Ann Surg 206:173–183
7. Bott S, Prakash C, MacCallum RW (1987) Medication-induced esophageal injury: survey of the literature. Am J Gastroenterol 82: 758–753

16   A. Quinton, F. Zerbib, and H. Lamouliatte

8. Bova JG, Dutton NE, Goldstein HM et al (1987) Medication-induced esophagitis: diagnosis by double-contrast esophagography. AJR 148: 731–732
9. Burrington JD (1975) Clinitest burns of the esophagus. Ann Thorac Surg 20: 400–404
10. Carlborg B, Densert O (1980) Esophageal lesions caused by orally administered drugs. An experimental study in the cat Eur Surg Res 12: 270–282
11. Carlborg B, Kumlien A, Olsson H (1978) Medikamentella esofagusstrikturer. Lakartidningen 75: 4609–4611
12. Channer KS, Virjee J (1982) Effect of posture and drink volume on the swallowing of capsules. Br Med J 285: 1702
13. Channer KS, Bell J, Virjee J (1984) Effect of left atrial size on the esophageal transit of capsules. Br Heart J 52: 223–227
14. Coates AG, Nostrandt TT, Wilson JA et al (1986) Esophagitis caused by nonsteroidal antiinflammatory medication: case reports and review of literature on pill-induced esophageal injury. South Med J 79: 1094–1097
15. Delpre G, Kadish U (1981) More on esophageal ulcerations due to tetracycline and doxycycline therapy. Gastrointest Endosc 27: 108–109
16. Delpre G, Kadish U, Stahl B (1989) Induction of esophageal injuries by doxycycline and other pills. A frequent but preventable occurrence. Dig Dis Sci 34: 797–800
17. Edwards P, Turner J, Gold J, Cooper DA (1990) Esophageal ulceration induces by zidovudine. Ann Intern Med 112: 65–66
18. Eichenberger P, Blum AL (1980) Drug-induced esophageal lesions. Acta Endosc 10: 273–278
19. Eng J, Sabanathan S (1991) Drug-induced esophagitis. Am J Gastroenterol 86: 1127–1133
20. Evans KT, Roberts GM (1976) Where do all tablets go? Lancet 2: 1237–1239
21. Florent C, Chagnon JP, Vivet P, Brun JG, Cattan D, Bernier JJ (1980) Accidents œsophagiens associés à la prise de doxycycline. Gastroenterol Clin Biol 4: 888–892
22. Giger M, Sonnenberg A, Brandli H, Singeisen M, Guller R, Blum AL (1978) Das Tetracyclin Ulkus der Speiseröhre. Dtsch Med Wochenschr 103: 1038–1040
23. Goff JS, Satterlee W (1985) Sucralfate and esophageal ulcers. Gastrointest Endosc 31: 50
24. Habeshaw T, Bennett JR (1972) Ulceration of mouth due to emepronium bromide. Lancet 1: 493
25. Heller SR, Fellows IW, Ogilvie AL, Atkinson M (1982) Nonsteroidal antiinflammatory drugs and benign esophageal stricture. Br Med J 285: 167–168
26. Hey H, Jorgensen F, Sorensen K, Hasselbach H, Warnberg T (1982) Esophageal transit of six commonly used tablets and capsules. Br Med J 285: 1717–1719
27. Kikendall JW, Friedman AC, Oyewole MA, Fleischer D, Johnson LF (1983) Pill-induced esophageal injury. Case reports and review of the medical literature. Dig Dis Sci 28: 174–182
28. Lauder AD (1979) Cetipirin and esophageal ulceration. Br Med J 2: 211
29. MacCall AJ (1975) Slow-K ulceration of esophagus with aneurysmal left atrium. Br Med J 3: 230–231
30. MacCord GS, Clouse RE (1990) Pill-induced esophageal strictures: clinical features and risk factors for development. Am J Med 88: 512–518
31. Minocha A, Greenbaum DS (1991) Pill-esophagitis caused by nonsteroidal antiinflammatory drugs. Am J Gastroenterol 86: 1086–1089
32. O'Meara TF (1980) A new endoscopic finding of tetracycline induced ulcers. Gastrointest Endosc 26: 106–107
33. Orr WC, Johnson LF, Robinson MG (1984) Effect of sleep on swallowing, esophageal peristalsis, and acid clearance. Gastroenterology 86: 814–819
34. Ovartlarnporn B, Kulwichit W, Hiranniramol S (1991) Medication-induced esophageal injury: report of 17 cases with endoscopic documentation. Am J Gastroenterol 86: 748–750

35. Papazian A, Capron JD, Dupas JL (1981) Doxycycline-induced esophageal ulcer. Value of Lugol's solution vital staining. Gastrointest Endosc 27: 201
36. Papazian A, Descombes P, Capron JP (1984) Œsophagite ulcéréé et mycotique après prise de Physiomycine. Gastroenterol Clin Biol 8: 389
37. Pemberton J (1970) Esophageal obstruction and ulceration caused by oral potassium therapy. Br Heart J 32: 267–268
38. Pilbrant A (1977) Ulceration due to emepronium bromide tablets. Lancet 1: 749
39. Pinos T, Figueras C, Mas R (1990) Doxycycline-induced esophagitis: treatment with liquid sucralfate. Am J Gastroenterol 85: 902–903
40. Rosenthal T, Adar R, Militanu J, Deutsch V (1974) Esophageal ulceration and oral potassium chloride ingestion. Chest 65: 463–465
41. Schreiber JB, Covington JA (1988) Aspirin-induced esophageal hemorrhage. JAMA 259: 1647–1648
42. Semble EL, Wu WC, Castell DO (1989) Nonsteroidal antiinflammatory drugs and esophageal injury. Semin Arthritis Rheum 19: 99–109
43. Spiller RC (1986) Where do all tablets go in 1986? Gut 27: 879–885
44. Williams JG (1979) Drug-induced esophageal injury. Br Med J 2: 273

NSAID Gastropathy

M. GUSLANDI

Gastroenterology Unit, S. Raffaele Hospital and Department of Biomedical Sciences, University of Milan, Italy

1 Epidemiological Data

Nonsteroidal anti-inflammatory drugs (NSAIDs) are among the most commonly prescribed drugs all over the world. In the United States the number of prescriptions is more than 100 million per year (for about 45 million patients), let alone another 40 billion aspirin tablets sold as over-the-counter drugs [2]. In the United Kingdom and in France the number of NSAID prescriptions reaches 23 million [15, 30].

NSAIDs are precious drugs but are unfortunately associated with various untowards effects, mainly on the digestive system and in particular the gastroduodenal tract. Gastrointestinal disorders by NSAIDs are the most common drug-induced adverse effects in the United States with 2600 deaths and 24,000 hospitalizations per year in patients with rheumatoid arthritis [16, 17]. The risk of hospitalization in NSAID users is up to 1.58 % per year, with a risk of death of 0.19 % per year [18]. According to a recent meta-analysis, the overall odds ratio of the risk for adverse GI events is 2.74 [19]. The risk appears to be dose-related [8] and has been found to be higher in subjects taking NSAID for less than 1 month or with concomitant use of corticosteroids [19, 25]. Elderly patients (who are the main consumers of NSAIDs) are particularly at risk. This might be due to a number of reasons: a reduced metabolization of the drugs with consequent increase in their toxicity, a higher mucosal vulnerability because of age-related atrophy, and a longer contact between NSAIDs and the gastric mucosa due to a delayed gastric emptying [65]. Dyspeptic symptoms during NSAID intake are reported in up to 60 % of patients [7, 75], 20 % of whom do not show any abnormalities at upper GI endoscopy [7, 15]. On the other hand, endoscopic injuries can be detected in percentages that in the some studies reach 74 % and 26 % of cases in the stomach and duodenum respectively.

Up to 76 % of NSAID gastropathies are symptomless [41], with consequent danger of sudden, unexpected massive bleeding. Again, elderly people, especially females, are particularly prone to develop asymptomatic gastric lesions [9]. Possible explanations for this phenomenon include the analgesic activity of NSAIDs and the subpopulation taking NSAIDs, since physicians may be reluctant to prescribe these drugs to dyspeptic subjects. NSAID-induced mucosal lesions are represented by erosions or ulcers. Gastric ulcers are five to ten times more frequent in NSAID users than in the normal population [21]. Occult, chronic microbleeding is extremely common, with the occurrence of iron deficiency anemia in up to 15 % of cases, but massive hemorrages are far from infrequent, with a mortality rate of 10 % or more [76].

An interesting question is whether the noxious effects of NSAIDs on the gastroduodenal mucosa is related to the type of anti-inflammatory drug. It is generally recognized that acetyl-salicylic acid (ASA) exerts damaging effects to a greater extent than other NSAIDs [7, 47]. The 24-h intake of aspirin induces gastric erosions in 90 % – 100 % of healthy volunteers and duodenal erosions in 50 % – 60 % [6, 73]. Yet, during chronic aspirin consumption the figures are reduced to 50 % and 17 %, respectively [7, 60], suggesting a mucosal adaptation to aspirin damage. Every attempt to rank the mucosal damaging activity among non-aspirin NSAIDs has failed due to different methodological approaches [6, 31, 73]. Conflicting results are reported, for instance, with drugs such as sulindac [6, 7] and piroxicam [54, 55, 73]. NSAIDs with nonacidic molecules may be less toxic (see below), but this must still be confirmed.

Multiple use of different NSAIDs or concomitant intake of steroids greatly increases the risk of developing NSAID gastropathy.

2 Mechanisms of NSAID Gastric Toxicity

It is now accepted that aspirin and other NSAIDs can damage the gastroduodenal mucosa through two main mechanisms [74]: a direct topical effect (which obviously takes place only after oral administration of the drug) and a systemic effect, after the drug is absorbed into the blood circulation, which is independent from the route of administration.

Furthermore, it has been suggested that NSAIDs can also act by means of a third mechanism, an indirect topical route, secondary to enterohepatic circulation of the drugs into the bile. Although this appears to be a major mechanism in NSAID small-bowel toxicity [3], it may also affect the gastric mucosa through duodenogastric bile reflux (Table 1).

Table 1. Mechanisms of NSAID gastropathy

Local (oral route)	Systemic (any route)
– Intracellular diffusion (acidic NSAIDs) – Direct damage to mucus and surface phospholipids – Direct inhibition of HCO_3 and blood flow	– Cyclo-oxygenase inhibition with defective prostaglandin production – Indirect impairment of mucus, HCO_3, and blood flow – Overproduction of lipo-oxygenase derivatives (leukotrienes) – Neutrophil adherence to vascular endothelium – Free radical production – Altered local ATP/AMP ratio

2.1 Direct Local Toxicity

Aspirin and most NSAIDs are weak organic acids which at gastric pH are usually nonionized. Therefore they are lipid soluble and diffuse freely through cellular membranes into the mucosal cells, where the higher pH induces acid dissociation. In the ionized state aspirin and acidic NSAIDs are water soluble and remain trapped inside the cell. This in turn leads to alterations in cell membrane permeability with back-diffusion of hydrogen ions from the lumen and subsequent mucosal damage [74]. The rate of absorption of aspirin is indeed dependent on intragastric pH, and aspirin-induced mucosal injury is reduced in achlorhydric patients and when gastric juice is buffered at pH 6–7 [38]. The topical damaging effect of aspirin seems to be important during acute administration, which is followed by an immediate drop in the gastric potential difference and extensive damage to the epithelial cells and the tight junctions [33, 64].

On the other hand, no significant alterations are detectable after a single parenteral dose of aspirin [40], whereas repeated administration results in mucosal damage, obviously by means of the systemic effect of the drug. Although impairment of mucosal defensive factors such as gastric mucus and bicarbonate secretion and local blood flow is thought to be related to inhibition of prostaglandin synthesis (see below), it is likely that to some extent these effects are due to a direct contact between NSAIDs and mucosa. For example, surface phospolipids are directly damaged by aspirin, with a consequent reduction in mucosal hydrophobicity [32].

2.2 Systemic Effects

Aspirin and NSAIDs are known to inhibit cyclo-oxygenase, which accounts for the development of gastroduodenal injury after administration by other routes than oral intake. The mucosa is usually protected against acid, pepsin, and noxious agents by a number of defensive factors, the first line of defense being the so-called mucus-bicarbonate barrier. The pH gradient between lumen and mucosa promotes back-diffusion of hydrogen ions. The viscous layer of mucus covering the gastric epithelium retards back-diffusing H^+ ions, thus promoting their neutralization by bicarbonate secreted into the mucus itself by the underlying cells. Hydrogen ions which have been able to escape the buffering activity of the barrier and to penetrate the mucosa are removed into the bloodstream by the local microcirculation, which also protects the mucosa by providing oxygen and nutrients.

Locally produced cytoprotective prostaglandins control the efficiency of the mucus-bicarbonate barrier by stimulating both production of mucosubstances and alkaline secretion and increase mucosal blood flow [28]. Inhibition of prostaglandin production obviously results in a breakdown of mucosal defences. However, the lack of correlation between the degree of prostaglandin inhibition by the various NSAIDs and their gastroduodenal toxicity [58, 59, 71] suggests that the importance of this phenomenon has probably been overestimated. In fact, it has been pointed out that cyclo-oxygenase inhibition not only reduces prostaglandin production but also shifts the synthetic activity toward lipo-oxygenase with a consequent increase in leukotriene production [70]. Leukotrienes are known to exert noxious effects on the gastric mucosa [26], and their antagonists have been found to decrease the gastric toxicity of indomethacin [70]. Furthermore, the increased lipo-oxygenase activity leads to a hyperproduction of free radicals with cytotoxic effects [59].

Recently a role for neutrophils in NSAID gastropathy has been proposed [83]. Neutrophil activation by NSAIDs (whether through a local or a systemic effect is not known) would result in their adherence to the vascular endothelium, with consequent reduced mucosal perfusion as well as release of tissue-damaging factors such as oxygen-derived free radicals. Other minor mechanisms that still await a full understanding include a reduction in ATP production and the ATP/AMP ratio which also induces oxyradical production through activation of xantine oxy dase [59]. Uncoupling of oxidative phosporylation by high doses of aspirin must be also borne in mind.

2.3 Other Noxious Mechanisms

The ability of aspirin and other NSAIDs to interfere with platelet function and to prolong bleeding time is certainly involved in promoting gastric bleeding once mucosal lesions are established [14]. A number of recent studies have demonstrated that NSAIDs exert unfavorable effects on epithelial repair, thus promoting and maintaining mucosal damage. Mucosal cell proliferation and DNA synthesis have been found to be markedly reduced during chronic NSAID administration [57, 66] as well as angiogenesis in the damaged tissues [37] with delayed healing of gastroduodenal erosions or ulcers [66, 77]. The above findings remain in apparent disagreement with the hypothesis that long-term adaptation to NSAID administration is related to increased cellular regeneration [22, 56]. The possibility that adaptation is due to an increase in intraluminal concentration of epidermal growth factor [42] warrants further evaluation.

A possible role of *Helicobacter pylori* in NSAID-induced peptic ulcers has been suggested [79], but the possibility that *H.pylori* infection influence the degree of mucosal damage associated with NSAID intake has been ruled out [23, 46, 61]. On the other hand, gastric mucosal injury and bleeding by NSAIDs seem to be more frequent in subjects without *H.pylori infection* [23], and the presence of the microorganism in the mucosa of chronic aspirin users is particularly low, a finding possibly related to the fact that in vitro the drug has bactericidal activity on *Helicobacter* in concentrations which are comparable to the plasma concentrations reached during therapy [8].

3 Prevention of NSAID Gastropathy

3.1 General Measures

Physicians should be aware that NSAIDs must be administered only if really necessary. When a mere analgesic effect is required (e. g., for treating headache), anti-inflammatory drugs, although effective, should be avoided, and paracetamol (acetaminophen) which is devoid of gastroduodenal toxicity [39, 44] should be prescribed. Concomitant administration of two or more NSAIDs increases the risk of gastric damage [7] and must be discouraged. The timing of drug intake could be also important: chronopharmacological studies in rats have shown, for instance, that the adverse gastric effects of aspirin are 50 % more severe if the drug is given in the evening compared with early morning [78]. Clearly, more studies are needed to acquire further information on this matter. It is generally advised to take aspirin and NSAIDs after eating in order to reduce the direct contact between the drug and the mucosa [78]. However, it has been shown in rats that mucosal injury by aspirin and indomethacin is more severe if the drugs are taken with food [10]. On the other hand, concomitant ingestion of alcoholic beverages is contraindicated since it may increase the gastric toxicity of NSAIDs [12].

On theoretical grounds, the choice of anti-inflammatory drug can also be important. NSAIDs with lower gastrointestinal toxicity should be preferred, but, as already mentioned, a ranking of their ability to promote mucosal injury is extremely difficult. Nonacidic drugs such as nabumetone and azapropazone may be less ulcerogenic in terms of direct, local effects [63], while NSAIDs with relatively scarce inhibitory activity on gastric cyclo-oxygenase, such as etodolac [50] and carpofen [43], may have a lower systemic gastric toxicity. In particular carpofen seems devoid of short-term adverse effects on the gastric mucosa not only in healthy volunteers [43, 50] but also in duodenal ulcer patients [44]. However, information on long-term gastroduodenal effects is still insufficient.

As already stated, the route of administration is of little consequence on the occurrence of NSAID gastropathy in that the systemic adverse effects of the drugs cannot be prevented [29, 48]. In the attempt to prevent a direct contact between NSAIDs and the gastric mucosa enteric-coated preparations have been developed. Enteric-coated aspirin appears to be less noxious to the gastric mucosa [34, 49, 69], but conflicting results are reported with naproxen [67, 81], and no significant advantages were observed with enteric formulations of ketoprophen [11].

The use of "buffered" aspirin does not seem to afford particular protection compared with the regular formulation [69, 35] (Table 2).

Table 2. Prevention of NSAID gastropathy. Theoretical general measures

- Use of paracetamol if only analgesic effects are required
- Avoid concomitant use of more than one NSAID or of NSAIDs plus steroids
- Intake of NSAIDs in the morning (?)
- Administration by nonoral route
- Buffered formulations of acidic NSAIDs
- Enteric-coated tablets

3.2 Pharmacological Prophylaxis

A large number of studies have addressed the problem of preventing NSAID gastropathy by coadministering a "protective" pharmacological agent, usually an anti-ulcer drug exerting acid-inhibiting effect or gastroprotective activity or both. There are two categories of studies: short-term experiments, mostly in healthy volunteers, testing the ability of the pharmacological agent to prevent mucosal damage and/or gastric bleeding induced either by a single dose of NSAID or by oral intake for a few days, and long-term trials where the possible prophylactic effect is determined in patients with rheumatologic disorders during continuous NSAID consumption for weeks or months.

3.2.1 Short-Term Studies

When administered 20–60 min before each dose of aspirin, given for periods of 1–12 days, all available ulcer-healing agents, whether antisecretory or gastroprotective, are significantly superior to placebo in reducing blood loss into the gastric juice [27]. Similarly, prostaglandin analogues either in antisecretory or cytoprotective doses, but not sucralfate, significantly decrease NSAID-induced fecal blood loss [27].

Endoscopic evaluations have been also performed, but employing different severity scores, which makes it hard to draw definitive conclusions. In the studies reporting rate of patients achieving total protection a normal gastric mucosal appearance was maintained in up to 45 % of cases with cimetidine, 66 % with sucralfate, and 73 % with misoprostol [27]. Superior results (which must be further confirmed) have been obtained with the proton pump inhibitor lansoprazole, which completely protects the gastric mucosa from damage by a single intake of 1 g aspirin in 92 % and 100 % of cases in doses of 30 mg and 60 mg, respectively [4]. In general, it appears that maintenance of a normal mucosa during short-term NSAID intake is easier in the duodenum, where even placebo can "protect" in 24 %–63 % of cases [27].

A significant reduction in the severity of the gastroduodenal endoscopic score in volunteers taking various NSAIDs has ben generally shown with acid inhibitors such as H_2 blockers, antacids in high doses, and omeprazole as well as with sucralfate and prostaglandin derivatives [27]. However, conflicting findings are also reported. Omeprazole 40 mg was found ineffective in preventing gastroduodenal lesions during a 2-week course of diclofenac [13]. Lanza et al. [51] pointed out that results may change substantially depending on the type of score used: both H_2 receptor antagonists and sucralfate appear unable to protect significantly from naproxen-induced gastroduodenal injury if only erosions and ulcers are taken into consideration, and petechial lesions are excluded from the analysis [51].

It is worth noting that prostaglandin derivatives appear to be equally active in high (i. e., antisecretory) and low (i. e., cytoprotective) doses. In particular, misoprostol 200 µg b. i. d. was found as effective as 200 µg q. i. d. in preventing gastroduodenal damage by aspirin, with a substantial decrease in the incidence of adverse intestinal events [53].

3.2.2 Long-Term Studies

Cimetidine proved to be significantly superior to placebo in reducing fecal blood loss during a 4-week administration of aspirin at 2.6 g daily, but no significant differences were observed in endoscopic and histological scores [85]. In contrast, a recent large study lasting 6 months disclosed a significant ability of the drug to reduce significantly the incidence of NSAID-induced peptic ulcers (6.9 % versus 15.7 % with placebo) [84].

Table 3. Controlled trials showing ranitidine superior to placebo in preventing NSAID-induced mucosal injury

Duration of treatment	Site of injury	
	Gastric	Duodenal
4 weeks	2/5 trials	2/4 trials
8 weeks	0/3 trials	2/3 trials

Various studies have been performed with ranitidine (Table 3), showing that the drug is able to decrease significantly the duodenal endoscopic score and to reduce the incidence of duodenal ulcer. A meta-analysis of the main double-blind, placebo-controlled trials confirmed that significantly fewer patients receiving ranitidine than placebo develop a duodenal ulcer during NSAID therapy [72]. In contrast, no significant protection by ranitidine is detectable in the stomach.

Misoprostol in antisecretory doses proved significantly better than placebo in preventing the development of gastric ulcers during a 3-month treatment with NSAIDs. Oddly, misoprostol failed to reduce the severity of dyspeptic symptoms, while diarrhea occurred in 39 % of cases [20]. In a similar study misoprostol proved to be significantly better than sucralfate, the incidence of gastric ulcers being 1.6 % and 16 %, respectively [1]. Recently, the effectiveness of misoprostol in the prevention of NSAID duodenal ulcers has also been confirmed by a multicenter, double-blind, placebo-controlled trial [24].

Favorable results in the prevention of gastric and duodenal injury by NSAIDs are also reported in double-blind, placebo-controlled trials with sulglycotide, a sulfated high molecular weight glycopeptide with gastroprotective activities [62,68] and able to prevent aspirin-induce inhibition of epithelial cell proliferation.

Coadministration of antiulcer agents and NSAIDs has raised the problem of possible interactions between the two classes of drugs, a problem which would be particularly important during long-term treatments. Aside from some minor interferences observed when using antacids or cimetidine, the therapeutic effect of NSAIDs is unhampered by concomitant use of antisecretory or gastroprotective drugs [27, 36].

4 Treatment of NSAID-Induced Gastroduodenal Lesions

In patients with NSAID-induced gastroduodenal injury who discontinue the anti-inflammatory treatment the standard therapeutic approach with H_2 blockers or sucralfate is equally effective as in subjects with erosions or ulcers unrelated to NSAID intake [27].

Unfortunately most patients on chronic NSAID therapy cannot stop the ongoing treatment because of their underlying rheumatologic disease. In these subjects both ulcers and erosions can be successfully treated with ranitidine, sucralfate, omeprazole, or antisecretory doses of misoprostol [27]. The results of controlled studies with cimetidine are inconclusive and in general disappointing [27].

Gastric ulcers tend to heal more slowly if NSAID therapy continues [5], a phenomenon which only omeprazole seems to overcome [82]. However, a recent multicenter trial has demonstrated that if treatment is prolonged to 12 weeks, the effectiveness of ranitidine 150 mg b.i.d. in healing gastric ulcers of patients still on NSAIDs reaches 79 %, a figure quite satisfactory, even though inferior to the healing rate obtained by the H_2 blocker if NSAIDs are stopped [46].

References

1. Agrawal N, Roth S, Graham DY, White RH, Germain B, Brown JA, Stromatt SC (1991) Misoprostol compared with sucralfate in the prevention of nonsteroidal anti-inflammatory drug-induced gastric ulcer. A randomized, controlled trial. Ann Intern Med 115: 195–200
2. Baum C, Kennedy DL, Forbes MB (1985) Utilization of nonsteroidal anti-inflammatory drugs. Arthr Rheum 28: 686–692
3. Beck WS, Schneider HT, Dietzel K, Nuernberg B, Brune K (1990) Gastrointestinal ulcerations induced by anti-inflammatory drugs in the rats. Physicochemical and biochemical factors involved. Arch Toxicol 64: 210–217
4. Bigard MA, Joubert M (1991) Prevention par le lansoprazole des lesiomnes gastriques induites chez le sujet sain par prise unique d'aspirine. Etude de doses. Gastroenterol. Clin Biol 15 (2 bis): A 122
5. Bjisma JW (1988) Treatment of NSAID-induced gastrointestinal lesions with cimetidine: an international multicentre collaborative study. Aliment Pharmacol Therap 2 (suppl 1): 85–96
6. Carson JL, Strome BL, Morse L (1987) The relative gastrointestinal toxicity of nonsteroidal antiinflammatory drugs. Arch Intern Med 147: 1054–1059
7. Caruso I, Bianchi Porro G (1980) Gastroscopic evaluation of anti-inflammatory agents. Br Med J 280: 75–78
8. Caselli M, Pazzi P, Lacorte R, Aleotti A, Trevisani L, Stabellini G (1989). Campylobacter-like organisms, nonsteroidal anti-inflammatory drugs and gastric lesions in patients with rheumathoid arthritis. Digestion 44: 101–104
9. Clinch D, Banerjee AK, Levy DW, Ostick G, Feracher EB (1987) Non-steroidal antiinflammatory drugs and peptic ulceration. JR Coll Physicians Lond 21: 183–187
10. Cole AT, Brundell S, Hudson N, Hawthorne AB, Mahida YR, Hawkey CJ (1991) Aspirin: take without food to limit gastric mucosal injury and with ranitidine to reduce bleeding? Gastroenterology 100: A 45

11. Collins AJ, Davis J, Dixon ASJ (1988) A prospective endoscopic study of the effects of Orudis and Oruvail on the super gastrointestinal tract in patients with osteoarthritis. Br J Rheumathol 27: 106–109

12. De Schepper PJ, Tjandramaga T, De Roo B (1978) Gastrointestinal blood loss after diflunisal and after aspirin: effect of ethanol Clin Pharmacol Ther 23: 669–676

13. Dorta G, Saraga E, Nicolet M, Schnegg JF, Vouillamoz D, Armstrong D, Blum AL (1991) Influence of omeprazole on healing and prevention of gastroduodenal mucosal lesions during administration of NSAIDs. Gastroenterology 100: A 55

14. Fellows IW, Bhaskar NK, Hawkey CJ (1989) Nature and time-course of piroxicam-induced injury to human gastric mucosa. Aliment Pharmacol Therap 3: 481–488

15. Florent C, Deasaint B (1989) Fréquence et gravité des lésions gastriques et duodénales induites par les anti-inflammatoires non stéroidiens et l'aspirine. Gastroenterol Clin Biol 13: 235–238

16. Fries JF (1988) Postmarketing drug surveillance: are our priorities right? J Rheumathol 15: 389–390

17. Fries JF, Miller SR, Spitz PW, Williams CA, Hubert HB, Bloch DA (1989) Toward an epidemiology of gastropathy associated with nonsteroidal antiinflammatory drug use. Gastroenterology 96: 647–655

18. Fries JF, Williams CA, Bloch DA, Michel BA (1991) Nonsteroidal anti-inflammatory drug-associated gastropathy: incidence and risk factors models. Am J Med 91: 213–222

19. Gabriel SE, Jaajjimainen L, Bombardier C (1991) Risk for serious gastrointestinal complications related to use of nonsteroidal anti-inflammatory drugs. Ann Intern Med 115: 787–796

20. Graham DY, Agrawal NM, Roth Sh (1988) Prevention of NSAID-induced gastric ulcer with misprostol: multicentre double-blind, placebo-controlled trial. Lancet II: 1277–1280

21. Graham DY, Lacey Smith J (1988) Gastroduodenal complications of chronic NSAID therapy. Am J Gastroenterol 83: 1081–1084

22. Graham DY, Lacey Smith J, Spjut HJ, Torres E (1988) Gastric adaptation. Studies in humans during continuous aspirin administration. Gastroenterology 95: 327–333

23. Graham DY, Lindski M, Cox AM, Evans DJ, Evans DG, Alpert L, Klein PD, Sessoms SL, Michaletz PA, Saeed ZA (1991) Long-term nonsteroidal antiinflammatory drug use and Helicobacter pylori infection. Gastroenterology 100: 1653–1657

24. Graham DY, Stromatt SC, Jaszewski R, White RH, Triadafilopoulos G (1991) Prevention of duodenal ulcer in arthritic who are chronic NSAID users: a multicenter trial of the role of misoprostol. Gastroenterology 100: A 75

25. Griffin MR, Piper JM, Daugherty JR, Snowden M, Ray WA (1991) Nonsteroidal anti-inflammatory drug use and increased risk for peptic ulcer disease in elderly persons. Ann Intern Med 114: 257–263

26. Guslandi M (1987) Gastric effects of leukotrienes. Prostagl Leukotr Med 26: 203–206

27. Guslandi M (1990) Pharmacological prevention and treatment of NSAID-induced gastroduodenal lesions. Drugs Today 26: 413–422

28. Guslandi M, Tittobello A (1991) Basic pathophysiology of gastric mucosal protection. In: Braga PC, Guslandi M, Tittobello A (eds) Drugs in gastroenterology. Raven, New York, pp 199–202

29. Hansen TN, Matzen P, Madsen P (1984) Endoscopic evaluation of the effect of indomethacin capsules and suppositories on the gastric mucosa in rheumathic patients. J Rheumathol 11: 484–487

30. Hazleman BL (1989) Incidence of gastropathy in destructive arthropathies. Scand J Rheumathol 78 (suppl): 1–4

31. Heller CA, Ingelfinger MD, Goldman P (1985) Nonsteroidal anti-inflammatory drugs and aspirin. Analyzing the scores. Pharmacotherapy 5: 30–38
32. Hill BA, Butler BD, Lichtenberger LM (1983) Gastric mucosal barrier: hydrophobic lining to the lumen of the stomach. Am J Physiol 7: G 561–G 568
33. Hingson D, Ito S (1971) Effect of aspirin and related compounds on the fine structure of mouse gastric mucosa. Gastroenterology 61: 156–177
34. Hoftiezer JW, Silvoso GR, Burks M, Ivey KJ (1980) Comparison of the effects of regular and enteric-coated aspirin on the gastroduodenal mucosa in man Lancet 2: 609–612
35. Hoftiezer JW, O'Laughlin JC, Ivey KJ (1982) Effects of 24 hours of aspirin, bufferin, paracetamol and placebo on normal human gastroduodenal mucosa. Gut 23: 692–697
36. Howden CW (1988) Review: interactions between H_2-antagonists and nonsteroidal anti-inflammatory drugs. Aliment Pharmacol Therap 2: 93–100
37. Hudson N, Balsitis M, Hawkey CI (1991) Reduction in angiogenesis in NSAID associated gastric ulcers. Gut 32: A 1246
38. Ivey KJ, Morrison S, Gray C (1972) Effects of salycilates on the gastric mucosal barrier in man. J Appl Physiol 33: 81–85
39. Ivey KJ, Silvoso G, Krause WJ (1978) Effect of paracetamol on human gastric mucosa. Br Med J 1: 1586–1588
40. Ivey KJ, Paone DB, Krause WJ (1980) Acute effect of systemic aspirin on gastric mucosa in man. Dig Dis Sci 25: 97–99
41. Jaszewski R (1990) Frequency of gastroduodenal lesions in asymptomatic patients on chronic aspirin or nonsteroidal antiinflammatory drug therapy. J Clin Gastroenterol 12: 10–13
42. Kelly SM, Dickinson RJ, Jenner JR, Hunter JO (1991) Gastric mucosal adaptation to continued non-steroidal anti-inflammatory drug administration: role of epidermal growth factor. Gut 32: A 58
43. Konturek SJ, Kwiecien N, Obtulowitz W (1982) Effect of carpofen and indomethacin on gastric function, mucosal integrity and generation of prostaglandins in man. Hepato-Gastroenterol 29: 267–270
44. Konturek SJ, Brzozowski T, Piastucki I, Radecki T (1982) Prevention of ethanol and aspirin-induced gastric mucosal lesions by paracetamol and salicylate in rats: role of endogenous prostaglandins. Gut 23: 536–540
45. Konturek SJ, Obtulowitz W, Kwiecien N (1984) Generation of prostaglandins in gastric mucosa in patients with peptic ulcer disease: effect of nonsteroidal antiinflammatory compounds. Scand J Gastroenterol 19 (suppl 101): 75–77
46. Lancaster-Smith MJ, Jaderberg ME, Jackson DA (1991) Ranitidine in the treatment of non-steroidal anti-inflammatory drug associated gastric and duodenal ulcers. Gut 32: 252–255
47. Lanza FL, Royer GL, Nelson RS, Chen TT, Seckman CE, Rack MF (1979) The effects of ibuprofen, indomethacin, aspirin, naproxen and placebo on the gastric mucosa of normal volunteers. Dig Dis Sci 24: 823–828
48. Lanza FL, Umbenhauer ER, Nelson RS, Rack MF, Daurio MS, White LA (1982) A double-blind randomized placebo controlled gastroscopic study to compare the effects of indomethacin capsules and suppositories on the gastric mucosa of helthy volunteers. J Rheumathol 9: 415–419
49. Lanza FL, Rack MF, Wagner GS, Balm TK (1985) Reduction in gastric mucosal hemorrhage and ulceration with chronic high-level qid and bid dosing of enteric coated aspirin granules. Dig Dis Sci 30: 509–512
50. Lanza FL, Panagides J, Salom IL (1986) Etodolac compared with aspirin: an endoscopic study of the gastrointestinal tracts of normal volunteers. J Rheumathol 13: 299–303
51. Lanza FL, Graham DY, Davis RE, Rack MF (1990) Endoscopic comparison of cimetidine and sucralfate for prevention of naproxen-induced acute gastroduodenal injury. Effect of scoring method. Dig Dis Sci 35: 1494–1499

52. Lanza FL, Evans DG, Graham DY (1991) Effect of Helicobacter pylori infection on the severity of gastroduodenal mucosal injury after the acute administration of naproxen or aspirin to normal volunteers. Am J Gastroenterol 86: 735–737

53. Lanza FL, Kochman RL, Geis GS, Rack EMF, Deysach LG (1991) A double-blind placebo controlled 6-day evaluation of two doses of misoprostol in gastro-duodenal mucosal protection against damage from aspirin and effect on bowel habits. Am J Gastroenterol 86: 1743–1748

54. Laporte JR, Carné X, Vidal X, Moreno V, Juan J (1991) Upper gastrointestinal bleeding in relation to previous use of analgesics and non-steroidal anti-inflammatory drugs. Lancet 337: 85–89

55. Larkai EN, Lacey Smith J, Lidsky MD, Sessoms SL, Graham DY (1989) Dyspepsia in NSAID users: the size of the problem J Clin Gastroenterol 11: 158–162

56. Levi S, Goodlad RA, Lee CY, Stamp G, Walport MJ, Wright NA, Hodgson HJF (1990) Inhibitory effect of non-steroidal anti-inflammatory drugs on mucosal cell proliferation associated with gastric ulcer healing. Lancet 336: 840–843

57. Levi S, Goodlad RA, Lee CY, Walport MJ, Wright NA, Hodgson HJF (1992) Effects of nonsteroidal anti-inflammatory drugs and misoprostol on gastroduo-denal epithelial proliferation in arthritis. Gastroenterology 102: 1605–1611

58. Levine RA, Petokas S, Nandi J, Enthoven D (1988) Effects of nonsteroidal anti-inflammatory drugs on gastrointestinal injury and prostanoid generation in healthy volunteers. Dig Dis Sci 33: 660–666

59. Ligumski M, Sestieri M, Karmeli F, Zimmerman J, Okon E, Rachmilewitz D (1990) Rectal administration of nonsteroidal antiinflammatory drugs. Effect of rat gastric ulcerogenicity and prostaglandin E2 synthesis. Gastroenterology 98: 1245–1249

60. Lockard O, Ivey KJ, Butt JH, Silvoso G, Sisjk C, Holt S (1980) The prevalence of duodenal lesions in patients with rheumatic disease on chronic aspirin therapy. Gastrointest Endosc 26: 5–72

61. Loeb DS, Talley NJ, Ahlquist DA, Carpenter HA, Zinsmeister AR (1992) Long-term nonsteroidal anti-inflammatory drug use and gastroduodenal injury: the role of Helicobacter pylori. Gastroenterology 102: 1899–1905

62. Loizzi P, D'Ingianna E, Ferri S (1990) Effectiveness of sulglycotide in prevention of gastric lesions by non-steroidal anti-inflammatory drugs in patients with rheu-mathic disease. A controlled double-blind endoscopic study vs placebo. Clin Trials J 27: 164–174

63. McCormack K, Brune K (1987) Classical absorption theory and the development of gastric mucosal damage associated with non-steroidal anti-inflammatory drugs. Arch Toxicol 60: 261–269

64. Meyer RA, McGinley D, Posalaky Z (1986) Effects of aspirin on tight junction structure of the canine gastric mucosa. Gastroenterology 91: 351–359

65. Moore JG, Bjorkman DJ (1988) NSAID-induced gastropathy, deaths and medieval practice. Ann Intern Med 109: 353–354

66. Myszor M, Hodgson HJF (1990) Non-steroidal anti-inflammatory drugs and gastric DNA synthesis. Scand J Gastroenterol 25: 197–202

67. Oddson E, Gudjonsson H, Thjodleifsson B (1990) Endoscopic findings in the stomach and duodenum after treatment with enteric-coated and plain naproxen tablets in healthy subjects. Scand J Gastroenterol 25: 231–234

68. Petrillo M, Bianchi Porro G, Ardizzone S (1991) Prevention of NSAID-induced gastrolesivity with sulglycotide. Hepato-Gastroenterol 38 (suppl): 45

69. Petroski D (1986) A comparison of enteric-coated aspirin granules with plain and buffered aspirin: a report of two studies. Am J Gastroenterol 81: 26–28

70. Rainsford KD (1988) Mechanisms of NSAID-induced gastrointestinal mucosal injury: a basis for preventing ulceration and symptoms for these agents. Aliment Pharmacol Therap 2 (suppl 1): 43–55

71. Rainsford KD, Willis C (1982) Relationship of gastric mucosal damage induced in pigs by anti-inflammatory drugs to their effect on prostaglandin production.

Dig Dis Sci 27: 624–635
72. Robinson M, Mills RJ, Euler AR (1991) Ranitidine prevents duodenal ulcers associated with non-steroidal anti-inflammatory drug therapy. Aliment Pharmacol Therap 5: 143–150
73. Rossi AD, Hsu JP, Falch GA (1987) Ulcerogenicity of piroxicam: an analysis of spontaneously reported data. Br Med J 294: 147–150
74. Schoen RT, Vender RJ (1989) Mechanisms of nonsteroidal anti-inflammatory drug-induced gastric damage. Am J Med 86: 449–458
75. Semble EL, Wu WC (1987) Antiinflammatory drugs and gastric mucosal damage. Semin Arthritis Rheum 16: 271–286
76. Silverstein FE, Feld AD, Gilbert DA (1981) Upper gastrointestinal tract bleeding. Predisposing factors, diagnosis and therapy. Arch Intern Med 141: 322–327
77. Stadler P, Armstrong D, Margalith D, Saraga E, Stolte M, Lualdi P, Mautone G, Blum AL (1991) Diclofenac delays healing of gastroduodenal mucosal lesions. Double-blind, placebo-controlled endoscopic study in healthy volunteers. Dig Dis Sci 36: 594–600
78. Szabo S, Spill WF, Rainsford KD (1989) Non-steroidal anti-inflammatory drug-induced gastropathy: mechanisms and management. Med Toxicol Adv Drug Exp 4: 77–94
79. Taha AS, Najhshabendi I, Lee FD, Sturrock RD, Russell RI (1992) Chemical gastritis and Helicobacter pylori related gastritis in patients receiving non-steroidal anti-inflammatory drugs: comparison and correlation with peptic ulceration. J Clin Pathol 45: 135–139
80. Tavares IA, Collins PO, Bennett A (1987) Inhibition of prostanoid synthesis by human gastric mucosa. Aliment Pharmacol Therap 1: 617–623
81. Tronstad RI, Aaland E, Holler T, Olaussen B (1985) Gastroscopic findings after treatment with enteric coated and plain naproxen tablets in healthy subjects. Scand J Gastroenterol 20: 239–242
82. Walan A, Bader JP, Classen M, Lamers CBHW, Piper DW, Rutgersson K, Eriksson S (1989) Effect of omeprazole and ranitidine on ulcer healing and relapse rates in patients with benign gastric ulcer. N Engl J Med 320: 69–75
83. Wallace JL 81992) Non-steroidal anti-inflammatory drug gastropathy and cytoprotection: pathogenesis and mechanisms re-examined. Scand J Gastroenterol 27 (suppl 192): 3–8
84. Wallin BA, Grier CE, Fox MJ, McCafferty JP, Wetherington JD, Palmer RH (1990) Prevention of NSAID-induced ulcers with cimetidine: results of a double-blind placebo controlled trial. Gastroenterology 98: A 146
85. Welsh RW, Bench HL, Harris SC (1978) Reduction of aspirin-induced gastrointestinal bleeding with cimetidine. Gastroenterology 74: 459–463

Steroid Ulcers

Z. Sandor and S. Szabo

Chemical Pathology Research Division, Dept. of Pathology, Brigham and Women's Hospital and Harvard Medical School, Boston, Massachusetts, USA

1 Introduction

"Steroid ulcer" is an unfortunate misnomer and clinical jargon because it implies a not clearly established relationship between steroids and ulcer. Neither of the words are actually being used very precisely: namely, steroid in this context usually means glucocorticoid while neglecting the modern classification of steroids (see below) and ulcer is not a precise definition either, because most of these lesions are actually superficial mucosal erosions and they rarely reach the stage of ulcer. Thus, first of all we would like to establish a few definitions and outline the scope of our review.

In this chapter the designation "steroid" is used as a group name of naturally occurring and synthetic hormones and their derivatives. The "ulcers" are mainly induced by certain corticoids, especially by glucocorticoids. "Erosion" is a superficial mucosal lesion which does not penetrate the muscularis mucosae while the ulcer is deep damage involving the muscularis propria.

Historically, the association between gastric erosions and ulcers and administration of glucocorticoids originates from the seminal observations in the 1930s of Hans Selye who first described of the phenomenon of biologic stress [67], namely, that stress as "the nonspecific response of the body to any demand made upon it" [76] is a complex interplay involving mainly the nervous and endocrine systems. This is essentially a defense reaction and adaptation although severe stress is often accompanied by pathologic changes.

The functional and structural alterations as described in the original historic papers and books of Selye [67, 74, 76] have been grouped into the "triad of stress" which involves (a) enlargement of the adrenal glands, (b) atrophy of the lymph nodes, thymus and spleen, as well as (c) erosions and ulcers in the gastrointestinal (GI) tract. The intensity of these changes varies in the stages of stress response (i.e., during the alarm reaction, adaptation and stage of exhaustion) and GI erosions and ulcers usually occur during the alarm reaction and the stage of exhaustion. The initial and subsequent research on biologic stress confirmed that during this neuroendocrine adaption changes also involve the activation of the adrenomedullary sympathetic nervous system and the hypothalamic hypophyseal – adrenocortical axis. This response is not specific from an etiologic point of view since many physical, chemical, biologic and psychologic agents can trigger hyperfunction of the neuroendocrine system and result in mucosal lesions in the GI tract [76, 80]. Since stress reaction involves not only the hypersecretion of glucocorticoids but also the release of epinephrine, norepinephrine and other neurotransmitters and hormones, the GI ulcers associated with stress are similar but not completely identical with glucocorticoid-induced ulcers. However, both glucocorticoids and catecholamines exert biphasic effect, i.e., large doses induce gastric erosions but in low doses they exert gastroprotection [41, 84].

The initial observations originating mostly from experimental animals, especially rats, have been corroborated by numerous case reports and clinical observations describing the development of gastric and duodenal ulcers in patients receiving large doses of glucocorticoids for the treatment of rheumatoid arthritis or other chronic inflammatory changes.

These observations were later confounded by new clinical reports and retrospective analysis which often doubted the development of "steroid ulcers" [30]. However, it was also revealed that patients receiving large doses of glucocorticoids were automatically given antacid or later on histamine (H_2) receptor antagonists to decrease gastric acidity and to antagonize the apparent ulcerogenic action of glucocorticoids [78].

From a research point of view the first animal experiments were also confounded by new findings demonstrating that low doses of glucocorticoids are important for the maintenance of integrity of the gastric mucosa since in adrenalectomized animals the standard gastroprotective ("cytoprotective") agents such as prostaglandins (PG) and sulphydryls (SH) loose their protective action which can be restored by replacement therapy with glucocorticoids but not mineralocorticoids [84]. Subsequent and parallel studies in other laboratories revealed that low doses of glucocorticoids essentially exert gastroprotection, e.g., prevent the development of acute gastric erosions induced by ethanol or indomethacin [16].

The association between steroids and GI ulcers was further complicated by the discovery of angiosteroids, which are naturally occurring and synthetic compounds which either exert angiostatic or angiogenic activity, i.e., inhibit or stimulate angiogenesis or new blood vessel formation, respectively [13, 81, 86]. Angiogenic steroids like peptides such as basic fibroblast growth factor (BFGF) which exert angiogenesis also demonstrate prominent ulcer healing properties, e.g., accelerate the healing of chronic duodenal ulcers induced by cysteamine [21, 79, 85]. The potent antiulcer effect of angiogenic steroids is not associated with decreased gastric acid secretion.

New studies performed by Hans Selye at the end of his scientific carrier revealed that pretreatment of rats with certain catatoxic steroids, but especially spironolactone, androgens and low doses of estrogens and glucocorticoids prevented the indomethacin-induced small intestinal ulcers [75]. This antiulcer effect of various steroids may only in part be ascribed to induction of hepatic drug-metabolizing enzymes and enhanced catabolism of toxicants (i.e., catatoxic effect). The other mechanisms of the antiulcerogenic action of steroids thus remain to be elucidated.

The major aim of this chapter is that following a brief review of the modern classification of steroids, we would like to review the development of GI ulcers after administration of glucocorticoids in experimental animals and patients. To clarify the frequent misunderstanding and misinterpretation of results and since some of the original observations (e.g., the gastroprotective properties of glucocorticoids and discovery of angiosteroids) originate from our laboratory, we also want to briefly describe the effect of steroids on ulcer prevention and healing.

2 Classification of Steroids

The first scientific classification of steroids was also described by Hans Selye [68, 69, 72]. The basis of this classification was the glandular origin of steroid hormones, i.e., steroids originating from the adrenal cortex were labelled corticoids while hormones synthesized in sex glands were called testoids, folliculoids, and luteoids [70, 72]. The latter groups were subsequently categorized as androgens, estrogens and progestogens (Table 1). Corticoids, which are more and more frequently being called corticosteroids, have been subdivided into gluco- and mineralocorticoids depending on their preferential effect on the metabolism of carbohydrates and minerals, respectively. It has also been known since the early 1940s that glucocorticoids exert an anti-inflammatory action, while the mineralocorticoids were found to be proinflammatory [71, 73, 74, 77].

Table 1. The classification of steroids and their effect on GI ulcers

Categories	Examples	Ulcer[a]		
		Induction	Prevention	Healing
Corticoids (corticosteroids)				
Glucocorticoids	Cortisol Dexamethasone Triamcinolone	+	+	+ −
Mineralocorticoids	DOC Aldosterone	?	−	?
Androgens	Testosterone	?	+	?
Estrogens	Estradiol Estrone	+[b]	+	?
Progestogens	Progesterone	+[b]	?	?
Angiosteroids				
Angiogenic steroids	Tetrahydro-S-21-Br Tetrahydro-S-21-I Cortisol-21-I Cortisone-21-I	−	?	+
Angiostatic steroids	11α-Epicortisol Cortexolone 17α-Hydroxy-progesterone Tetrahydro S	+	?	−

+, Positive effect or stimulation;
−, negative effect or inhibition;
?, no (definitive) data are available; DOC, desoxycorticosterone
[a] "Ulcer" usually refers to gastric erosions and ulcers, unless otherwise stated.
[b] Lesions in the small intestine and colon.

Some of these steroids, but especially glucocorticoids, exert biphasic effects: PG and certain other so-called gastroprotective agents and mediators of inflammation may induce or aggravate lesions in the

GI tract but in low doses they often exert gastroprotective actions [82, 86]. Glucocorticoids in high doses may also cause gastric erosions and ulcers in experimental animals but in low doses these hormones are essential for gastroprotection [16, 84].

The angiotropic agents or angiosteroids discovered to be related to a new target organ, i. e., angiogenesis, have also been incorporated into Table 1. Just as the anesthetic property of certain steroids [68] is often shared with an other biologic effect (e. g., progesterone), the angiotropic action of steroids is also an independent but often shared steroid effect, e. g., both the glucocorticoid and antiglucocorticoid cortisol and 11α-epicortisol as well as the hormonally inactive cortexolone inhibit the development of new blood vessels in the presence of heparin [13, 20, 81]. Furthermore, like the effect of ulcerogenesis, the action of cortisol and certain other steroids on angiogenesis is biphasic, and this might be the reason, at least partially, for the ulcerogenic and antiulcerogenic effect of certain glucocorticoids (see below).

The effect of steroids on GI ulcers is also listed in Table 1. since like other steroids which exert antiulcerogenic action, angiogenic steroids accelerate the healing of experimental chronic duodenal ulcers [86].

3 Animal Experiments

The possibility that corticoids have a role in the development of stress-induced gastric erosions and ulcers was considered from the 1940s and 1950s, when the concept of biologic stress was described. To test this hypothesis numerous experiments using mostly large doses of corticoids were performed [54, 56].

3.1 Gastric Ulcers

The early studies in rats and mice demonstrated that gastric injury (i. e., erosions and ulcers) readily develop after administration of multiple doses of glucocorticoids injected mainly subcutaneously to fasted animals. These experiments also revealed that the new synthetic and more potent glucocorticoids were more ulcerogenic than the naturally occurring cortisol (Table 2). Furthermore, the relative ulcerogenic and glucocorticoid potencies of natural and synthetic glucocorticoids seemed to run parallel (Table 2). The ulcerogenic potencies of cortisol, prednisolone and 6α-methylprednisolone is also similar to their relative anti-inflammatory action. Triamcinolone and dexamethasone are, on the other hand, about 4–11 times more ulcerogenic than 6α-methylprednisolone, which is about eight times less anti-inflammatory than triamcinolone, while dexamethasone is about 17 times more potent an anti-inflammatory drug than 6α-methylprednisolone. Thus, the ulcerogenic property of glucocorticoids shows good correlation with their effect on glycogen metabolism and their anti-inflammatory effect. These correlations will be further analyzed below when discussing the pathogenesis of GI ulceration.

Table 2. Relative ulcerogenic properties of glucocorticoids in comparison with their effect on hepatic glycogen deposition and anti-inflammatory potency (from [2])

Corticoids	Relative ulcerogenic potency	Relative glucocorticoid potency	Relative anti-inflammatory potency
Hydrocortisone (cortisol)	1.0	1.0	1.0
Prednisolone	2.5	5.0	2.7
6α-Methylprednisone	8.0	13.0	6.0
Triamcinolone	30.0	108.0	48.5
Dexamethasone	87.0	90.4	104.0

The induction of gastric erosions and ulcers by cortisol and synthetic glucocorticoids as described by Robert et al. [55] and Wallace [88] is summarized in Table 3. In these studies fasted rats were injected subcutaneously once daily between 8.00 and 9.00 a.m. for 4–6 consecutive days with cortisol (10 mg), prednisolone (50 mg/kg), or dexamethasone (4 mg/kg) sodium phosphate.

Table 3. Methods of inducing experimental gastric erosions and ulcers in the rat

Glucocorticoids	Dose	Route of administration	Dosage
Cortisol	10 mg	Subcutaneous	once per day for 4 days
Prednisolone (prednisolone-21-sodium succinate)	50 mg/kg	Subcutaneous	once per day for 6 days
Dexamethasone (dexamethasone sodium phosphate)	4 mg/kg	Subcutaneous	once per day for 6 days

The results showed that the corticosteroids caused multiple gastric erosions and ulcers in time and partially dose-dependent manner [54, 56]. After 1 or 2 days of glucocorticoid administration gastric lesions were not detected, but after 4 days of dexamethasone injection gastric damage was observed. By the sixth day both dexamethasone and prednisolone further increased ($p < 0.001$) the damage score. In all the parameters at all time intervals dexamethasone was clearly much more ulcerogenic than prednisolone. The dose dependency of ulcer induction by dexamethasone was more apparent than of prednisolone [88]: namely, when 10, 50, or 100 mg/kg prednisolone was injected to the rats subcutaneously once daily for 6 days, the two lower doses of the steroid caused similar gastric damage and the highest dose did not further enhance the gastric injury.

The erosions and ulcers developed mainly in the acid-producing glandular part of the stomach, e. g., mostly in the corpus, rarely in the antrum, and the duodenum was not affected [55, 57]. The lesions appeared mainly as extensive, uniform hyperemia with focal regions of hemorrhage. These so called steroid-induced ulcers were usually superficial and healed rapidly. Histologically the main characteristic of these lesions usually were: focal necrosis and loss of the mucosa with crater formation, very little inflammatory reaction when the lesion was limited to the mucosa but severe inflammation when it reached the submucosa. Perforation usually did not occur in these experiments.

Cortisone acetate may cause gastric ulcer in non-fasted rats also, but only after 3 weeks administration in higher doses. Corticoids in animal experiments were shown to delay gastric ulcer healing [32], cause enlargement of experimental ulcers, and induce recurrence of previously healed ulcers [33].

Antisecretory compounds (e. g., methscopolamine bromide) [52], as well as PGE1 [9], PGE2 [61], and 16,16-dimethyl PGE2 [50, 61] were beneficial. Growth hormone given to hypophysectomized animals has the same effect [59]. The very potent dexamethasone was found to prevent the acute GI mucosal injury induced by platelet-activating factor [89].

3.2 Intestinal Ulcers

In addition to gastric ulcers some nonsteroidal anti-inflammatory drugs (NSAID) such as indomethacin induce ulcers in the jejunum and ileum as well. These small intestinal ulcers produced by daily subcutaneous injection of indomethacin were prevented by pretreatment of rats not only with catatoxic steroids such as spironolactone, pregnenolone-16α carbonitrile (PCN) and anabolic androgens but also by small doses of estrogens or glucocorticoids, such as prednisolone and triamcinolone [75]. This surprising antiulcer effect of small doses of glucocorticoids can be demonstrated not only macroscopically but by light microscopic histologic examination as well [75].

Multiple and large doses of glucocorticoids on the other hand, induce erosions and ulcers in the small intestines of rodents. Lancaster and Robert investigated the damaging effect of prednisolone on the rat small intestines [38]. Prednisolone injected subcutaneously at a dose of 10 mg, once a day for 8 days induced multiple necrotic lesions and often perforated ulcers mainly in terminal ileum and occasionally in the lower jejunum. The early lesions detected at 5 days were localized in the mucosa, then progressed towards the serosal side and often the whole thickness of intestinal wall became necrotic and infiltrated with polymorphonuclear leukocytes. The cecum and colon were very rarely affected. Very often bacterial colonies were visible on the surface of the lesions. Oral administration of antibiotics (e. g., neomycin, bacitracin and polymyxin B) prevented the development of ulcers, although the antibiotics had no effect on the concomitantly developed gastric ulcers. Thus, bacteria seem to play a role in the development of prednisolone-induced small intestinal ulcers.

Glucocorticoids and NSAID may induce ulcers in the stomach, jejunum and ileum, but never in the duodenum of small experimental animals. Duodenal ulcers, which is the most frequent form of human "peptic ulcer", may be experimentally induced only by specific duodenal ulcerogens such as cysteamine [25, 79, 83]. It was recently discovered that oral treatment with angiogenic steroids (Tables 1, 4) accelerated the healing of chronic cysteamine-induced duodenal ulcers in rats [86]. This potent antiulcerogenic effect of certain steroids was not associated with inhibition of gastric secretion but may be related to the ability of angiogenic steroids to stimulate angiogenesis, granulation tissue production, and other wound healing properties.

4 Clinical Experience

Clinicians usually held that "steroids" (i. e., glucocorticoids) cause peptic (i. e., gastric and duodenal) ulcers. In reality, however, the ulcerogenic effect of these drugs in patients is not clear [30] as a large amount of controversial data, mostly 10–30 years old, exist. These are mainly poorly documented studies performed before the introduction of endoscopic examination in patients receiving small or large doses of glucocorticoids, very often concomitantly with other drugs, including antacids and antisecretory agents [78].

4.1 Glucocorticoids

The first large retrospective analysis of clinical studies on the side effect of corticoids was published on in 1976 [11]. This involved 26 double-blind, prospective, controlled investigations with 3558 cases and

Table 4. The antiulcer potency of steroids in the cysteamine-induced chronic duodenal ulcer model in rats

Group	Steroid	Dose (mg/100g)	Antiulcer potency (max.: 100)
1	Cortisol	0.1	4.3
2	Cortisol	1.0	57.7
3	Cortisol	10.0	35.3
4	11α-Epicortisol	0.1	38.0
5	11α-Epicortisol	1.0	19.4
6	Progesterone	10.0	49.2
7	Cortisone-21-I	1.0	43.5
8	Cortisone-21-Br	1.0	46.2
9	Cortisol-21-Tosylate	1.0	59.8
10	Cortisol-21-I	1.0	32.7
11	Tetrahydro-S-21-Br	1.0	83.6

[a]The anti-ulcer potency was calculated as the arithmetic mean of the percent decrease in duodenal ulcer size and percent decrease in ulcer incidence for each steroid at every dose tested. The results are pooled from several experiments performed in our laboratory and are presented in part in [65].

demonstrated no significant difference in peptic ulcer occurrence between placebo and glucocorticoid groups (Table 5).

In this study peptic ulcer developed in 1.0 % of the 1491 control subjects and in 1.4 % of the 2067 glucocorticoid-treated patients, statistically, this difference was not significant. In addition 16 prospective, controlled, but not double-blind investigations, which included 1773 additional cases, were also analyzed. The not double-blind group showed a slight increase in occurrence of peptic ulcer in corticoid-treated patients, but the difference was not statistically significant. The final results based on the analysis of all the 42 studies with 5331 patients demonstrated that corticoids increase the risk of development of GI ulcers only in patients who had been taking the drug for more than 1 month or in high doses equivalent of 1000 mg of prednisone [11].

The large amount of data collected and published by Conn et al. [11] were analyzed again by Messer et al. in 1983 (Table 5). This second interpretation of data resulted in opposite conclusions on 3064 steroid-treated patients. Among these patients 55 (1.8 %) had ulcers, compared with 23 of 2897 controls (0.8 %) (relative risk 2.3, 95 % confidence interval 1.4–3.7). This increase from about 1 % to 2 % suggests that corti-

Table 5. The ulcerogenic properties of glucocorticoids in recent major clinical studies

Authors and year	Type of study	patients (n)		Conclusions (ulcers and corticoids)
Conn et al. [11]	Analysis of 26 prospective double-blind and 16 prospective, non- double-blind studies	2067 1491 918 855	Treated Controls Treated Controls	No correlation, except after 1 month duration and/or above 1000 mg prednisone
Messer et al. [40]	"Controlled clinical trial"	3064 2897	Treated Controls	Increased risk of peptic ulcer
Poynard [47]	Meta-analysis of randomized double- blind trials	3335 3267	Treated Controls	No significant correlation but "weak cause – effect relationship cannot be excluded"
Niwa et al. [42]	Retrospective	150	Treated	Correlation but only in patients with hypoalbuminemia
Piper et al. [45]	Retrospective case control	1415	Treated	Corticoids double the risk of peptic ulcers (from 1% to 2%) when coadministered with NSAID. Estimated relative risk: 14.6%

coids modestly increase the incidence of peptic ulcer. GI hemorrhage was especially more frequent in the glucocorticoid-treated group: 78 of 3135 steroid-treated patients (2.5%) had bleeding as compared with 48 of 2976 controls (1.6%) (relative risk 1.5, 95% confidence interval 1.1–2.2). The incidence of GI ulcers was directly related to the dosage of glucocorticoids. Messer et al. "strongly suggested" that corticoids do increase the risk of peptic ulcers and GI hemorrhage. The fault in Conn's study apparently was the acceptance of the null hypothesis (non association between steroids and peptic ulcer; type 2 error) followed by the misinterpretation of the absence of statistically significant correlation between steroid treatment and ulcer development. The other difficulty was that neither the first nor the second study was prospective, resulting in variable criterias.

In 1990 Poynard performed a meta-analysis of all published randomized, double-blind clinical trials comparing corticoids and placebo (Table 5). The prevalence of peptic ulcer was 0.4% in the steroid group ($n = 3335$) and 0.3% in the placebo group ($n = 3267$) : the difference statistically not significant. Poynard, however, also suggested that although a "weak cause – effect relationship cannot be absolutely" excluded, it is not necessary in practice to prescribe preventive antiulcer drugs to all patients receiving corticoids [47].

The prevalence of the adverse effects of corticosteroids in asthmatics was analyzed in another study [17]. The average length of use of prednisolone was 5.3 years; the mean dose was 26.2 mg every second day, in 85 patients. The prevalence of hypertension, peptic ulcer disease, pathologic fractures was not significantly increased over the normal population [17].

The ulcer-inducing effect of corticoids was examined in the study by Niwa et al. [42] in 150 patients with rheumatoid arthritis (RA) and with systemic lupus erythematosis (SLE). Marked hypoalbuminemia was found in the RA patients and this hypoalbuminemia showed significant statistical correlation with the incidence of peptic ulcer, which was especially elevated in patients with both hypoalbuminemia and corticoid administration [42]. A positive correlation between the incidence of GI ulcers in RA patients and the activity of the inflammatory disease was also documented.

In NSAID users the estimated relative risk for peptic ulcer disease for current, intermediate or former oral corticoid users was 4.4 (95 % confidence interval 2.0 to 9.7), 1.8 (confidence interval: 0.9 to 3.6) and 0.9 (confidence interval: 0.6 to 1.4). In the cortisol group not using NSAID there was no increased risk for GI ulcers associated with any category of oral corticoid use. However, in current steroid users who were also receiving NSAID the estimated relative risk for development of ulcer disease increased in relation with dose and duration. These results showed that the use of oral corticoids doubled the risk for peptic ulcer (estimated relative risk 2.0, 95 % confidence interval 1.3–3.1), while in patients using corticoids and NSAID at the same time had an estimated relative risk of 14.6 (confidence interval: 6.7–32), compared with those who used neither drug [45]. From the clinical point of view, then, glucocorticoids and NSAID should not be prescribed at the same time. If this combination of drugs is given, a very high risk of ulcer development is likely, and, for patients receiving long-term corticoids, coadministration of gastroprotective agents (e. g., misoprostol, sucralfate) should be considered [30].

4.2 Other Steroids

Only very limited data are available concerning the GI ulcerogenic effects of steroids other than glucocorticoids. Estrogens and progesterone cause mainly intestinal, but not gastric injury in humans. This adverse effect, however, is poorly investigated and the only study originates from the time of introduction of oral contraceptive drugs. Oral contraceptives and drugs containing estrogens and progesterone may cause ischemic lesions in the GI tract – mainly in the small intestines and colon [6, 12, 31, 36, 87]. Ischemic lesions are the result of thrombosis in mesenteric arteries or veins, leading to segmental hemorrhage, infarcts and ischemic enteritis [24, 49, 87].

5 Pathogenesis of Steroid Ulcers

Several hypotheses have been developed to understand the pathogenesis of glucocorticoid-induced gastric lesions. It is really unclear whether glucocorticoids cause gastric mucosal damage both in experimental animals and humans or predispose the mucosa to damage induced by other drugs, and/or interfere with the repair of existing damage. There is no doubt that glucocorticoids can induce acute erosions and ulcers in laboratory animals if given long enough and at high enough doses [43, 54]. Similar action of glucocorticoid in humans have been suggested, but the latest data are controversial. Thus most of the pathogenic results reviewed below originate from animal experiments.

5.1 Effect on Gastric Acid Secretion

One of the earliest explanations of steroid ulcers was the observation that corticoids elevate acid secretion not only in dogs [7, 8, 10, 27, 46, 48] but in humans, too [27]. The number of parietal cells increased when glucocorticoid were administered to experimental animals [10, 19, 48]. These results, however, originate from experiments of very long corticoid treatment.

Continuous administration of cortisone in dogs increased the G-cell population by 237 % compared to controls, and markedly elevated antral mucosal gastrin concentration to 370 % of control values [14]. The authors suggested that glucocorticoids play an important trophic role for antral gastrin cells.

Despite these data, originating mostly from animal experiments, the etiologic role of enhanced gastric acidity by corticoids in ulcer development is questionable: namely, gastric acid hypersecretion caused by corticoids is not very pronounced and very potent secretagogues such as pentagastrin do not cause gastric ulcers in animals. Infusion of pentagastrin and histamine in rats, on the other hand, induces duodenal ulcers or erosions which are usually associated with hyperacidity. In patients acid hypersecretion is mainly characteristic of duodenal ulcer and not of gastric ulcer, which is the most frequent localization of lesions after corticoid administration and which leaves acidity in the stomach either normal or even diminished. Additional controversial data originate from animal experiments: prednisolone administration in ulcerogenic doses in rats markedly reduced gastric acid secretion and output [51].

Thus enhanced gastric acidity plays a small or only contributory role in the pathogenesis of gastric ulceration induced by glucocorticoids.

5.2 Glucocorticoid and the Mucus – Bicarbonate Barrier

Corticoids were found to abolish the increased gastric alkaline secretion caused by noxious stimuli in rats, but they have no effect on duodenal bicarbonate secretion [23, 44].

Decreased mucus production by corticoids might also have a role in gastric ulceration. The effect on mucus secretion may develop directly through the inhibition of gastric mucus synthesis or through the effects of glucocorticoids on cell turnover. These actions were observed both in dogs [39] and in rats [39, 53, 56].

Both adherent and soluble mucus were decreased in the gastric juice and mucosa after continuous administration of prednisone for several weeks [29]. The diminished mucus was observed before the ulcer developed, suggesting that the low mucus concentration might have been the reason for ulcer development. The reduced production of mucus was detected by S-35 incorporation, indicating a decrease in the synthesis of sulfated mucoproteins [15, 34].

5.3 Influence on Prostaglandin Synthesis

The possible inhibition of synthesis of PG, which usually exert protection in the stomach, might be on additional reason for ulcer development after long-term treatment with glucocorticoids. Indeed, corticoids in experimental animals reduced the activity of phospholipase A1, which catalyzes the liberation of PG precursor arachidonic acid from phospholipids [88].

An additional specific mechanism in the pathogenesis of GI ulceration might be the fact that certain PG increase mucus synthesis in the stomach of dogs [3, 5], rats [4], and humans [22, 64, 65]. One of the first experiments performed in rabbits and guinea pigs demonstrated that corticoids inhibited the release of PG in perfused mesenteric blood vessels and perfused lungs [28]. This inhibitory effect is believed to be mediated by the proteins lipocortins [18].

Since PG exert certain "cytoprotective" effects on the gastric mucosa [51, 62, 63], it was a logical postulate [38, 44, 66] that the reduction of the PG release by corticoids may lead to gastric injury and might be a pathway in their ulcerogenic action. Experiments performed by Wallace, however, showed that the glucocorticoid-induced gastric damage was not accompanied by either elevation or reduction of gastric PG levels as measured by 6-keto $PGF1\alpha$ concentration in the rat gastric fundus. The conclusion of two previous experiments [9, 90] has also been that PG synthesis in the rat gastric mucosa is not inhibited by glucocorticoids. Thus, it is controversial and unlikely that PG depletion may have a role in the pathogenesis of corticoid-induced gastric mucosal injury.

5.4 Effect on Leukotrienes and Neutrophilic Myeloperoxidase

To examine the effect of corticoids on the leukotrienes (LT) and PG synthesis [88], dexamethasone and prednisolone in ulcerogenic doses were used in rats. Both corticoids markedly reduced gastric LTC4 synthesis, but dexamethasone was more effective than prednisolone. Short, i. e., 6-h administration of dexamethasone or prednisolone did not show significant effect on LTC4 synthesis. Administration of prednisolone for 2–6 days caused a 40 %–60 % reduction in gastric LTC4 levels, which was not significant. Dexamethasone given for 2–6 days, however, decreased gastric LTC4 synthesis by $>90\%$ ($p < 0.001$) and reduced gastric and other tissue levels of the neutrophilic enzyme myeloperoxidase. There was a highly significant ($p < 0.001$) correlation between the inhibition of LT synthesis and the reduction of gastric tissue level of neutrophilic myeloperoxidase.

It is not clear whether the effects of glucocorticoids on gastric LTC4 synthesis and myeloperoxidase activity are relevant to the pathogenesis of gastric ulceration induced by these steroids [88]. These actions on the other hand, might be part of the mechanism of mucosal protection and anti-inflammatory action by glucocorticoids [2, 16, 84].

5.5 Opportunistic Infections

The prolonged use of corticoids often predisposes to the development of opportunistic infections of the GI tract. The appearance of bacteria and viruses in the stomach may have a role in the pathogenesis of gastritis and peptic ulcer disease [26]. For instance consumption of steroids may predispose to H. pylori positivity in the stomach, providing hence an additional mechanism for chronic inflammation, ulceration and/or lack of appropriate healing in the stomach and duodenum.

5.6 "Stress Ulcers" vs. "Steroid Ulcers"

Gastric ulcers induced by glucocorticoid administration and those developing during severe stress are different entities, although they may share some pathogenic features. Stress ulcers after severe trauma and during other severe illness and shock etc. can develop even after adrenalectomy [57]. Gastric erosions and ulcers induced by stress are detectable within a few hours but in animal experiments corticoids must be given for days to produce gastric ulcers. Under stress, the blood level of glucocorticoid is elevated, but apparently higher levels are needed for the development of gastric ulcer [57]. In addition, during severe stress numerous other pathogenetic changes may play a role in ulceration, e. g., vasoconstriction, reduced blood flow and elevated secretion of catecholamines and other neurotransmitters.

The final pathway of gastric ulceration induced by glucocorticoids in experimental animals is still poorly understood despite intensive research during the past decades. We attempted to summarize the likely pathogenic events in Table 6, but we are afraid that we have to put more emphasis on the need for new investigations rather than to delineate a common pathway of glucocorticoid-induced gastric ulceration.

Table 6. Possible pathogenetic pathways of gastric mucosal damage induced by glucocorticoids

Glucocorticoids
→   Enhanced gastric acid secretion (?)
    G cell hyperplasia
    Increased of gastrin secretion
    Elevated number of parietal cells
→   Interference with inreased gastric alkaline
    Secretion caused by noxious stimuli
→   Decreased mucus production
    (Adherent and soluble)
→   Reduction of PG synthesis (?)
→   Reduction of cell turnover
→   Inhibition of angiogenesis
→   Development of opportunistic infection especially bacterial colonization

Nevertheless, it appears that the ability of glucocorticoids to cause gastric erosions and ulcers is in good correlation with their effect on glycogen deposition in the liver (Fig. 1) and their anti-inflammatory potency (Fig. 2). Beyond that, enhanced gastric acid secretion is an unlikely pathologic event, while diminshed alkaline secretion in response to injury, decreased mucus secretion, and cell turnover, as well as inhibition of angiogenesis by glucocorticoids seem to represent the major common pathogenic factors in this type of gastric ulceration.

6 Conclusion

After the modern classification of steroids into corticoids (gluco- and mineralocorticoids), androgens, estrogens, progestogens and angiosteroids (angiogenic and angiostatic steroids) as well as review of animal experiments and clinical data on GI ulcer induction, prevention and healing by steroids, it becomes clear that (a) large and multiple doses of

GC potency

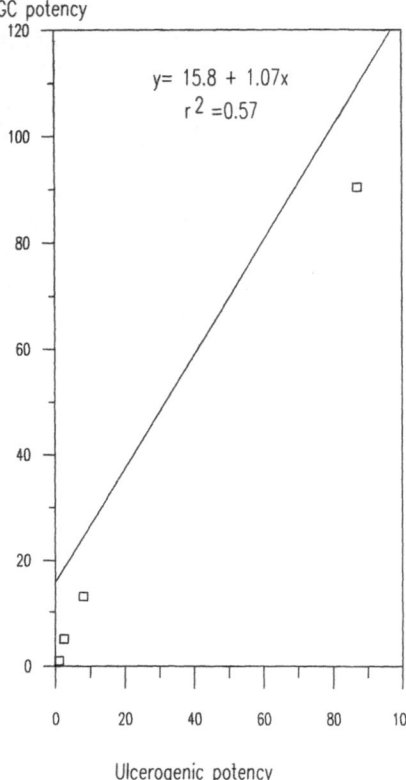

Ulcerogenic potency

Fig. 1. Correlation between glucocorticoid *(GC)* and ulcerogenic potencies of corticoids. (From [2])

glucocorticoids invariably induce erosions and ulcers in the stomach, less frequently in the jejunum and ileum of experimental animals, (b) the ability of gastric ulcer induction by corticosteroids is proportional to their glucocorticoid and anti-inflammatory potency, (c) small doses of glucocorticoids, androgens and estrogens prevent the chemically induced acute mucosal lesions in the stomach and small intestine, (d) circulating glucocorticoids but not mineralocorticoids are essential for the manifestation of gastroprotection by PG and SH compounds, and (e) treatment with novel angiogenic steroids accelerated the healing of experimental chronic duodenal ulcers in rats without inhibition of gastric secretion. Clinical observations demonstrate that estrogens and progestogens may induce small intestinal ulcers, while the ability of glucocorticoids to cause "peptic", i.e., gastric and duodenal ulcers, has been confounded by the frequent, parallel intake of antacids or antisecretory drugs. Nevertheless, it appears that the ulcerogenic side effect of standard doses of glucocorticoids clinically is minimal, unless these steroids are administered with NSAID or accompanied by hypoalbuminemia. The pathogenesis of GI ulceration caused by glucocorticoids is

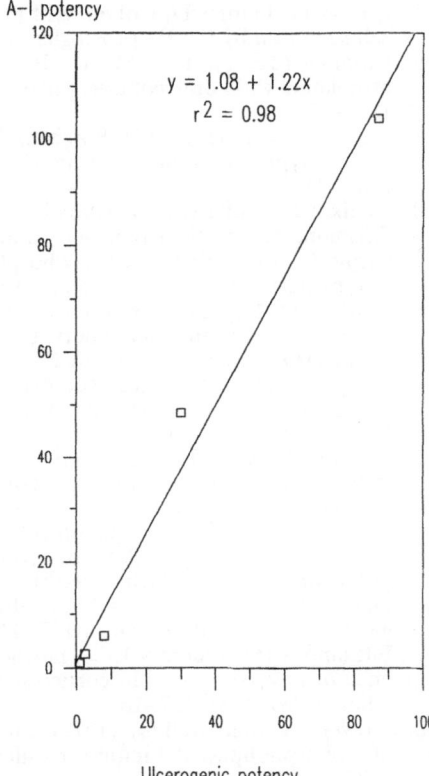

Fig. 2. Correlation between anti-inflammatory *(A-I)* and ulcerogenic potencies of corticoids. (From [2])

poorly understood. Gastric acid hypersecretion and PG depletion play a minimal or no role, while diminished alkaline and mucus secretion, decreased cell turnover, and inhibition of angiogenesis are probably the common ulcerogenic factors. The biphasic nature of action of glucocorticoids and the poorly understood ulcerogenic and antiulcerogenic effects of some steroids warrant further need for both basic and clinical investigations.

References

1. Bernandino ME, Lawson TL (1976) Discrete colonic ulcers associated with oral contraceptives. Dig Dis Sci 21: 503–506
2. Briggs MH, Brotherton J (1970) Steroid biochemistry and pharmacology. Academic, Press, London
3. Bolton JP, Cohen MM (1978) Stimulation of non-parietal cell secretion in canine Heidenhain pouches by 16,16-dimethyl prostaglandin E2. Digestion 17: 291–299
4. Bolton JP, Palmer D, Cohen MM (1976) Effect of the E2 prostaglandins on gastric mucus production in rats. Surg Forum 1976; 27: 402–403

5. Bolton JP, Palmer D, Cohen MM (1978) Stimulation of mucus and nonparietal cell secretion by the E2 prostaglandins. Am J Dig Dis23: 359–364
6. Brennan MF, Clarke AM, MacBeth WAAG (1969) Infarction of the midgut associated with oral contraceptives: report of two cases. N Engl J Med279: 1213–1214
7. Carbone JV, Leibowitz D, Forsham P (1957) Suppression of prednisone-induced gastric hypersecretion by an anticholinergic drug. Proc Soc Exp Biol Med94: 293–294
8. Chaikof L, Janke WH, Pesaros PC, Ponka JL, Brush BE (1961) Effect of prednisolone and corticotropin secretion. Arch Surg83: 32–46
9. Cirino G, Sorrentino L (1986) Phospholipase inhibition and prostacyclin generation by gastric muscularis and mucosa layers. Agents Actions18: 535
10. Clarke SD, Neill DW, Welbourn RB (1960) The effects of corticotropin and corticoids on secretion from denervated gastric pouches on dogs. Gut1: 36–43
11. Conn HO, Blitzer BL (1976) Nonassociation of adrenocorticosteroid therapy and peptic ulcer. N Engl J Med294: (9) 473–479
12. Cotton PB, Thomas ML (1971) Ischemic colitis and the contraceptive pill Br Med J3: 27–28
13. Crum R, Szabo S, Folkman J (1985) A new class of steroids inhibits angiogenesis in the presence of heparin or heparin fragment. Science 230: 1375–1378
14. Delaney JP, Michel HM, Bonsack ME, Eisenberg MM, Dunn DH (1978) Adrenal corticosteroids cause gastrin cell hyperplasia. Gastroenterology76: 913–916
15. Denko CW (1958) The effect of hydrocortisone and cortisone on fixation of S35 in the stomach. J Lab Clin Med51: 174–177
16. Derelanko MJ, Long JF (1982) Influence of prednisolone on ethanol-induced gastric injury in rat Dig Dis Sci27: 149–154
17. Fitzsimons R, Grammer LC, Halwig JM, Aksamit T, Patterson L (1988) Prevalence of adverse effects in corticosteroid dependent asthmatics. New Engl Reg Allergy Proc9 (2): 157–162
18. Flower RJ, Blackwell GJ (1979) Anti-inflammatory steroids induce biosynthesis of a phospholipase A2 inhibitor which prevents prostaglandin generation. Nature278: 456
19. Foley WA, Glick D (1962) Studies on histochemistry: LXVI. Histamine, mast and parietal cells in stomach of rats and effects of cortisone treatment. Gastroenterology43: 425–429
20. Folkman J, Ingber DE (1987) Angiostatic steroids. Ann Surg206 (3): 374–383
21. Folkman J, Szabo S, Stovroff N, McNeil P, Li W, Shing Y (1991) Duodenal ulcer: discovery of a new mechanism and development of angiogenic therapy that accelerates healing. Ann Surg214: 414–426
22. Fung WP, Lee SK, Karim SMM (1974) Effect of prostaglandin 15(R)-15-methyl E2-methyl ester on the gastric mucosa in patients with peptic ulcer action. An endoscopic and histologic study. Prostaglandins5: 465–472
23. Garner A, Heylinds JR, Hampson SE, Stanier AM (1990) Pharmacological profile of duodenal alkaline secretion. Alimentary Pharmacol. Ther4: 465–476
24. Gelfand MD (1972) Ischemic colitis associated with a depot synthetic progesterone. Dig Dis Sci17: 275–277
25. Giampaolo C, Gray AT, Olshen RA, Szabo S (1991) Predicting chemically induced duodenal ulcer and adrenal necrosis with classification trees. Proc Natl Acad Sci88: 6298–6302
26. Goldman H, Szabo S (1992) Chemical and physical disorders. In: Ming SC, Goldman H (eds) Pathology of the gastrointestinal tract. Saunders, Philadelphia; pp141–170
27. Gray SJ, Ramsey CG, Villereal R, Krakauer LJ (1955) Adrenal influences upon the stomach and the gastric response to stress. In: Selye, H, Heuser G (eds) Fifth annual report on stress 1955–1956; Acta Inc Med Publishers. Montreal, pp138–160

28. Gryglewski R J, Panczenko B, Korbut R Grrodzinska L, Ocetiwicz A (1975) Corticosteroids inhibit prostaglandin release from perfused mesenteric blood vessels of rabbit and from perfused lungs of sensitized guinea pigs. Prostaglandins 10: 343–355
29. Guslandi M (1990) Gastric mucus. In: Scarpignato C, Bianchi Porro G (eds) Clinical investigation of gastric function. Karger, Basel, pp 103-126
30. Guslandi M, Tittobello A (1992) Steroid ulcers: a myth revisited. B M J 304: 655–656
31. Hoyle M, Kennedy A, Prior A L et al. (1977) Small bowel Ischaemia and infarction in young women taking oral contraceptives and progestational agents. Br J Surg 64: 533–537
32. Janowitz H D, Weinstein V A, Shaer R G, Cereghini J F, Hollander F (1958) The effect of cortisone and corticotropin on the healing of gastric ulcer: an experimental study. Gastroenterology 34: 11–20
33. Kahn D S, Phillips M J, Skoryna S C (1961) Healed experimental gastric ulcer in rat: reulceration resulting from cortisone administration. Arch Pathol 38: 177–187
34. Kawarada Y, Lambek J, Matsumoto T (1975) Pathophysiology of stress ulcer and its prevention II. Prostaglandin E 1 and microcirculatory responses in stress ulcer. Am J Surg 129: 217–222
35. Kelly P, Robert A (1969) Inhibition by pregnancy and lactation of steroid induced ulcers in rat. Gastroenterology 56: 24–29
36. Kilpatrick Z M, Silverman J F, Betancourt E et al (1968) Vasvular occlusion of the colon and oral contraceptives. N Engl J Med 278: 438–440
37. Kuroiwa M, Sugiyama S, Tsukamoto Y, Goto H, Ohara A, Hosoino H et al. (1991) Effect of NSAIDs and steroids on healing of ethanol-induced gastric lesions in rats: steroids are not noxious agents against gastric injury. Gastroenterology 100: A 102
38. Lancester C, Robert A (1978) Intestinal lesions produced by prednisolone: prevention (cytoprotection) by 16,16-dimethyl prostaglandin E2. Am J Physiol 235: E 703
39. Menguy R, Masters Y F (1963) Effect of cortisone on mucoprotein secretion by gastric antrum of dogs: pathogenesis of steroid ulcer. Surgery 54: 19–28
40. Messer J, Reitman D, Sacks H S, Smith H, Chalmers T C (1983) Association of corticosteroid therapy and peptic ulcer disease. N Engl J Med 309: 21–24
41. Mozsik Gy, Suto G, Vincze A, Zsoldos T (1987) Correlation between free radicals and membrane-dependent energy systems in ethanol-induced gastric mucosal damage in rats. In: Szabo S, Pfeiffer C J (eds) Ulcer disease. CRC, Boca Raton, pp 15–29
42. Niwa Y, Iio A, Niwa G, Sakane T, Tsunematsu T, Kanoh T (1990) Serum albumin metabolism in rheumatic diseases: relationship to corticosteroids and peptic ulcer. J Clin Lab Immunol 31: 11–16
43. Nobuhara Y, Ueki S, Takeuchi K (1985) Influence of prednisolone on gastric alkaline response in rat stomach. A possible explanation for steroid-induced gastric lesion. Dig Dis Sci 30: 1166
44. Nobuhara Y, Ueki S, Takeuchi K et al. (1985) Influence of prednisolone on gastric alkaline response in rat stomach. Dig Dis Sci 30: 1166–1173
45. Piper J M, Ray W A, Daughterty J R Griffin M R (1991) Corticosteroid use and peptic ulcer disease: role of nonsteroidal anti-inflammatory drugs. Ann Int Med 114: 735–740
46. Plainos T C, Niktopulu G K, Vudykis P K (1962) The effect of triamcinolone and dexamethasone on gastric secretion and the excretion of uropepsin tested in dogs. Gastroenterology 43: 448–456
47. Poynard T (1990) Critical study of gastroduodenal complications of corticotherapy. Rev Practicien 40: 553–555
48. Reid N C, Hackett R M, Welbourn R B (1961) The influence of cortisone on the parietal cell population of the stomach in the dog. Gut 2: 119–122

49. Rhodes JM, Cockel R, Allan RN et al. (1984) Colonic Crohn's disease and use of oral contraception. B M J 288: 595–596
50. Robert A (1973) Prostaglandins and the digestive system. In Prostaglandines. INSERM, Paris, pp 297–315
51. Robert A (1979) Cytoprotection by prostaglandins, Gastroenterology 77: 761–767
52. Robert A, Nezamis JE (1959) Prevention of steroid-induced ulcers with an anti-cholinergic drug. Proc Soc Exp Biol Med 100: 596–597
53. Robert A, Nezamis JE (1963) Effect of prednisolone on gastric mucus content and ulcer formation. Proc Soc Exp Biol Med 114: 545–550
54. Robert A, Nezamis JE (1963) Ulcerogenic property of steroids. Proc Soc Exp Biol Med 114: 545–550
55. Robert A, Nezamis JE (1964) Effect of an anti-acetylcholine drug, methscopolamine bromide on ulcer formation and gastric mucus. J Pharm Pharmacol 16: 690–695
56. Robert A, Nezamis JE (1964) Histopathology of steroid induced ulcers. An experimental study in the rat Arch Pathol 77: 407–423
57. Robert A, Szabo S (1983) Stress ulcers. In: Selye H (ed) Selye's guide to stress research. Scientific and Academic Edition 2: 22–46
58. Robert A, Phillips JP, Nezamis JE (1966) Prevention of ulcer formation by hypophysectomy. Proc Soc Exp Biol Med 121: 992–995
59. Robert A, Phillips JP, Nezamis JE (1966) Gastric secretion and ulcer formation after hypophysectomy and administration of somatotrophic hormone. Am J Dig Dis 11: 516–522
60. Robert A, Nezamis JE, Phillips JP (1968) Effect of prostaglandin E 1 on gastric secretion and ulcer formation in the rat. Gastroenterology 55: 481–487
61. Robert A, Schultz JR, Nezamis JE, Lancester C (1976) Gastric antisecretory and antiulcer properties of PGE2, 15-methyl PGE2, and 16,16-dimethyl PGE2. Intravenous, oral and intrajejunal administration. Gastroenterology 70: 359–370
62. Robert A, Nezamis JE, Lancester C, Hanchar AJ (1977) Gastric cytoprotective property of prostaglandins. Gastroenterology 72: 1121
63. Robert A, Nezamis JE, Lancester C, Hanchar AJ (1979) Cytoprotection by prostaglandins in rats: prevention of gastric necrosis by alcohol, HCl, NaOH, hypertonic NaCl and thermal injury. Gastroenterology 77: 433–443
64. Ruppin H, Person B, Domschke W et al. (1979) Zytoprotektive Wirkungen von Prostaglandin E2 auf die Magenschleimhaut beim Menschen. Dtsch Med Wochenschr 104: 1457–1458
65. Ruppin H, Person B, Robert A et al. (1979) Gastric cytoprotection by prostaglandins (PG): possible medication by mucus secretion. Physiologist 22: 110
66. Scott J (1981) Physiological, pharmacological and pathological actions of glucocorticoids on the digestive system. Clin Gastroenterol 10: 62
67. Selye H (1936) A syndrome produced by diverse nocuous agents. Nature 138: 32
68. Selye H (1941) Anesthetic effect of steroid hormones. Proc Soc Exp Biol Med 46: 116–121
69. Selye H (1941) Pharmacological classification of steroid hormones. Nature 148: 84–85
70. Selye H (1942) Correlation between the chemical structure and the pharmacological actions of the steroids. 30: 437–453
71. Selye H (1942) Production of nephrosclerosis by overdosage with desoxycorticosterone acetate. Can Med Ass J 47: 515–519
72. Selye H (1943) An attempt at a natural classification of the steroids. Nature 151: 662–667
73. Selye H (1944) Role of the hypophysis in the pathogenesis of the diseases of adaptation. 50: 426–433
74. Selye H (1950) Stress. Montreal Acta, Inc, Montreal
75. Selye H (1971) Hormones and resistance. Springer, New York
76. Selye H (1976) Stress in health and disease. Butterworths, Boston

77. Selye H, Dosne C (1940) Treatment of wound shock with corticosterone. Lancet 2: 70
78. Spiro HM (1983) Is steroid ulcer a myth? N Engl J Med 309: 405–407
79. Szabo S (1978) Animal model of human disease: duodenal ulcer disease; animal model: cysteamine-induced acute and chronic duodenal ulcer in rat Am J Pathol 93: 273–276
80. Szabo S (1980) Stress and gastroduodenal ulcers. Stress 1: (2) 25–36
81. Szabo S (1985) The antiangiogenic activity of hydrocortisone is independent of its glucocorticoid activity. In: Folkman J (ed) Toward an understanding of angiogenesis: search and dicovery. Perspect Biol Med 29: 29
82. Szabo S (1991) Mechanisms of gastric mucosal injury and protection. J Clin Gastroenterol 13 [Suppl 2]: S 21–S 34
83. Szabo S, Cho CH (1988) From cysteamine to MPTP: structure-activity studies with duodenal ulcerogens. Toxicol Pathol 16: 205–212
84. Szabo S, Gallagher GT, Horner HC, Frankel PV, Underwood RH, Kontwoek SJ et al. (1983) Role of adrenal cortex in gastric mucosal protection by prostaglandins, sulfhydryls and cimetidine in the rat. Gastroenterology 85: 1384–1390
85. Szabo S, Vattay P, Morales RE (1989) Orally administered bFGF mutein: effect on healing of chronic duodenal ulcers in rats. Dig Dis Sci 34: 1323
86. Szabo S, Vattay P, Morales RE, Saha B, Neumayer JL, Lequesne PW (1991) Effect of a new class of steroids on healing of experimental chronic duodenal ulcers. Gastroenterology 100: A 171
87. Tedesco FJ, Volpicelli NA, Moore FS (1982) Estrogen- and progesterone-associated colitis: a disorder with clinical and endoscopic features mimicking Crohn's colitis. Gastrointest Endosc 28: 247–249
88. Wallace JL (1987) Glucocorticoid-induced gastric mucosal damage: Inhibition of leukotriene, but not prostaglandin biosynthesis. Prostaglandins 34: 311–323
89. Wallace JL, Whittle BJR (1988) Gastrointestinal damage induced by platelet-activating factor. Inhibition by corticoid dexamethasone. Dig Dis Sci 33: 225–232
90. Whittle BJR (1978) Potential endogenous inhibitor of prostaglandin synthetase in plasma: failure to inhibit cyclo-oxygenase in platelets and gastric mucosa. J Pharm Pharmacol 30: 467

Gastric Motility Disturbances by Drugs

T. K. Chaudhuri, S. Fink, and S. K. Wilson

Veterans Affairs Medical Center, Hampton, Virginia 23667, USA

1 Introduction

A major consequence of drug-induced changes in gastric motility is the effect on the rate of gastric emptying (GE). Drugs are one of many factors affecting GE. The characteristics of the gastric contents are a major factor, including its volume, size, density, temperature, viscosity, osmolality, and caloric value. Splanchnic blood flow, body position, and electrolyte balance also affect GE. Even gravity (or its absence) plays a role in the rate of GE [2]. The presence of food generally delays GE.

The nature of ingested food can affect GE directly and can also trigger delayed intestinal inhibition of GE of solids. Ingested carbohydrates may escape proximal absorption, travel over time to reach intestinal inhibitory mechanisms, and slow the GE of a later meal [67]. This factor combined with the diversity of meals, drugs, and rate of gastrointestinal (GI) drug absorption makes it difficult to separate the effect of a drug from concurrently ingested food [112]. In this chapter it is therefore understood that the effects of oral medication upon gastric motility are based upon studies in which the medication was ingested without rather than with meals.

Our review focuses primarily upon man but includes observations in other species. In addition to compounds foreign to the body we include the effect upon GE of endogenous compounds which are also administered therapeutically,.

2 Prescribed Drugs Affecting Gastric Emptying

2.1 Cardiovascular Drugs

Medications used to treat hypertension and heart disease are widely used. Supplemental potassium, often prescribed in conjunction with diuretics, tends to delay GE. This major cation of intracellular fluid is a factor in many physiologic processes, including transmission of nerve impulses and contraction of smooth muscle. Solutions containing potassium salts delay GE, leaving the stomach more slowly than does plain water [51, 79].

Intravenously administered dopamine slows the emptying of fasting gastric contents [78] and related L-dopa, given orally, delays the emptying of a mixed solid-liquid meal [7]. The calcium-channel blocking drugs used in the treatment of hypertensive and ischemic cardiovascular disease appear to have little effect upon GE. One evaluation of the effect of nifedipine on GE [8] found an increase in liquid transit time which was slight and statistically nonsignificant. Several studies using liquid and solid markers [100, 111] found no effect of nifedipine on GE of either component. Finally, a study using a semisolid meal in 11 men with a mean age of 60 years did show a delay after 20 mg oral nifedipine, with a mean GE half-time of 63.7 min compared to 42 min after placebo (Figs. 1, 2, Tables 1–4) [15–17, 34, 41]. Reviewing the data from these studies and noting that aging is more likely to be associated with delayed GE of liquids than of solids [76, 108], it has been suggested that clinicians remain aware of possible delayed GE in elderly patients taking semisolid or liquid diets whose therapeutic regimen includes nifedipine [15].

The anorexia, nausea and vomiting caused by cardiac glycosides are at least partially mediated by the area postrema of the medulla, and there is no evidence for a direct effect of these agents upon gastric motility. Nausea and vomiting are common adverse reactions to quinidine. These symptoms occur even when drug concentrations in plasma are low and are more likely due to gastric irritation than a consistent direct physiologic gastric effect. Beta-adrenergic blocking drugs such as propanolol and atenolol may also cause nausea which appears unrelated to a direct effect upon gastric motility. Phenytoin and procainamide exhibit antiarrhythmic properties similar to those of quinidine and may also cause nausea and vomiting. These reactions, less common than with quinidine, are also believed to reflect local gastric irritation.

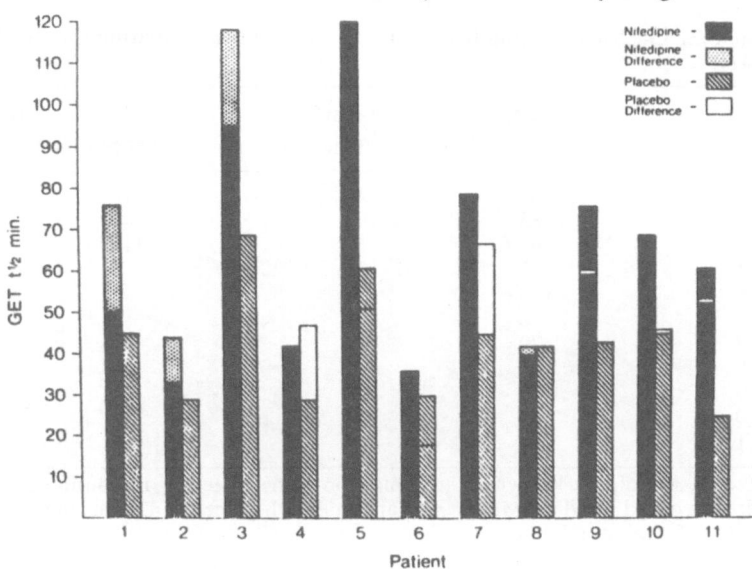

Fig.1. Effect of nifedipine on GE half-time *(GET ½)*; differences in 11 patients comparing placebo with nifedipine and the effect of placing nifedipine or placebo in test sequence. The place of nifedipine or placebo in the test sequence did not affect the data. (Reproduced with permission from [41])

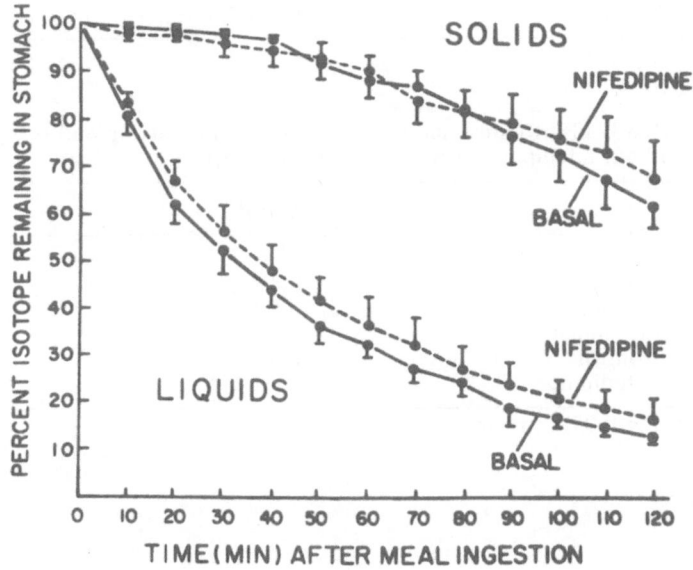

Fig.2. Effect of nifedipine on gastric emptying of liquid (water) and solid (chicken liver). Note no significant difference in gastric emptying between basal and nifedipine for either liquid or solid components. (Reproduced with permission from [111])

Table 1. Gastric emptying half-times for 11 patients comparing the three tests (from [41])

Patient no.	Test 1 Nifedipine	Test 2 Placebo	Test 3	
			Nifedipine	Placebo
1	50	45	76	
2	33	29	44	
3	95	69	118	
4	42	29		47
5	120+	61		51
6	36	30		18
7	79	45		67
8	40	42	42	
9	76	43	60	
10	69	45		46
11	61	25	53	

Test 1, nifedipine known; test 2, placebo known; test 3, nifedipine or placebo randomized and blinded. Mean GE half-time with placebo, 42 min; mean GE half-time with nifedipine, 63.7 min.

Table 2. Gastric emptying with and without nifedipine (30 mg per os) (from [100])

	Liquid	*Solid*
Control	11.5 ± 1.7	47 ± 4.0
Nifedipine	10.0 ± 2.0	35 ± 3.4

Table 3. Gastrointestinal motility index during fasting and postprandially with and without nifedipine (30 mg per os; from [100])

	Antral
Fasting	
Control	144 ± 27
Nifedipine	$65 \pm 19*$
Postprandial	
Control	194 ± 61
Nifedipine	$37 \pm 17*$

* $P < 0.05$, compared to controls.

Table 4. Gastric emptying rates with and without nifedipine (20 mg; from [8])

Study	Control group (5)			
	Liquid marker emptied in 10 min (%)	Half-time liquid marker (min)	Solid marker emptied in 10 min (%)	Solid marker emptied per min (%)
Placebo	11.8 ± 3.1	39.5 ± 6.8	6.5 ±1.8	0.31 ±0.1
Nifedipine	15.0 ± 5.8	43.0 ± 7.0	9.9 ±2.8	0.28 ±0.13

2.2 Respiratory Drugs

Beta-adrenergic drugs are first-line drugs in the treatment of asthma, combining bronchodilating activity with usually acceptable side effects. Beta-adrenergic agonists such as isoproterenol have been shown to delay GE of a mixed solid-liquid meal [96], an effect which is blocked by propanolol. Theophylline and other xanthines are also used for their ability to induce bronchial smooth muscle relaxation. The xanthines have been shown to cause relaxaton of the lower esophageal sphincter and stimulate gastric secretion (without change in serum gastrin levels), so that gastroesophageal reflux may complicate therapy [60]. However the effect of therapeutic levels of these drugs upon GE is not yet established. Although the anticholinergic agents are among the oldest of all respiratory drugs, they have rarely been used in recent years. It is possible that newer derivatives such as ipratropium will have a role in the alleviation of bronchospasm, in which case their ability to delay GE could assume therapeutic significance [115].

2.3 Gastrointestinal Drugs

Atropine, belladonna, and hyoscyamine are natural examples of the antimuscarinics which competitively inhibit the muscarinic effects of acetylcholine. By their action on autonomic effectors innervated by postganglionic cholinergic nerves and to a lesser extent on smooth muscles that lack cholinergic innervation, these compounds cause muscular relaxation and inhibit gastric motility. As a result, delayed GE follows oral as well as parenteral administration of most anticholinergic compounds [9, 18a, 27, 42, 52, 56], including the newer antimuscarinics such as propantheline [81]. Cimetropium bromide, a new antimuscarinic drug (also a quarternary ammonium compound) used for long-term treatment of irritable bowel syndrome, has spasmolytic activity on the esophagus, colon, and gall bladder but little or no effect on gastric motility [56]. Parenteral administration of the synthetic antimuscarinic glycopyrrolate is followed by a delaying effect on GE which does not follow oral administration [19]. The delaying effect upon GE by atropine appears to be greater in elderly than in younger subjects [95].

Ganglionic blocking drugs such as hexamethonium [32, 42] also slow gastric motility. Slowing by the antimuscarinics does not involve this mechanism since cholinergic transmission at autonomic ganglia involves nicotinic as well as muscarinic activity, with the result that even high doses of the antimuscarinics cause only partial ganglionic block.

Aluminum ion causes a gastric retention which greatly exceeds that observed after atropine [79]. Studies using the double isotope technique [90] demonstrated that one gram of the aluminum-containing compound sucralfate (190 mg aluminum) delayed GE of both liquid (water) and solid (chicken liver mixed with beef stew) meal components in duodenal ulcer patients but had no effect on GE in normal subjects. Another study [70] also using the dual isotope technique did not show a change in GE after sucralfate but demonstrated a slowing effect on GE of solids by therapeutic doses of an aluminum-containing antacid. The difference appears to be related to the amount of aluminum in the two therapeutic regimens, with GE delay attributable to the greater amount of aluminum delivered via the antacid gel [70].

Histamine delays GE of solid food in man, a delay prevented by administration of histamine H_1-antagonists. The role of H_2 receptors in regulation of gastric motility is less clear. It appears that cimetidine does not alter the rate of GE in man [68, 102, 103], but ranitidine causes delayed GE of solids [104] and intravenous ranitidine can also affect GE of liquids [21]. One report [102] mentions different effects of cimetidine and ranitidine on GE in rats and man. In rats, cimetidine in low doses does not have any effect on GE, whereas it significantly delayed GE in high doses. Ranitidine always accelerates GE in rats. In contrast, in humans, ranitidine delays GE and cimetidine has no effect in either low or high doses (Fig. 3).

In monkeys an intravenous infusion of cimetidine at doses capable of completely suppressing intragastric acidity slows GE [29] and the specific H_2 receptor agonist dimaprit increases GE [31]. This could suggest that histamine H_2 receptors are involved in the regulation of GE in man, but this conclusion is not fully accepted at this time [103]. Possible species differences, the anticholinergic effects observed in rats with very high doses of H_2 antagonists, and possible nonspecific effects in different species related to the individual H_2 antagonists all complicate interpretation of the animal data.

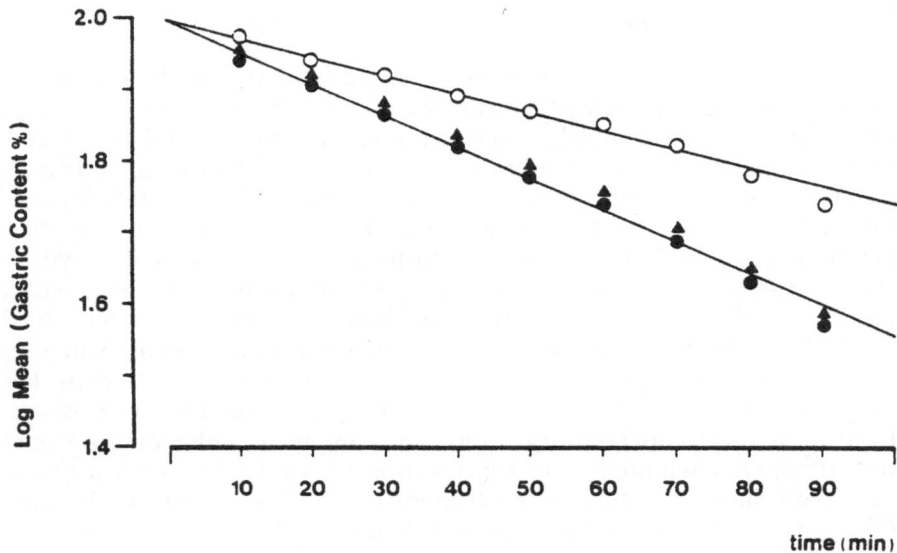

Fig. 3. Effect of cimetidine (▲) and ranitidine (○) on GE time in man (●, control). Note that cimetidine has no effect, and that ranitidine delays GE time. (Reproduced with permission from [102])

2.4 Endocrine Drugs

Estrogen and progesterone appear to have delaying effects upon GE [23, 24] and GI transit [113]. Menstruating women (particularly in luteal phase when progesterone levels are increased) have slower GE than postmenopausal women [24, 53, 55, 98], and both premenopausal women and postmenopausal women taking sex hormone replacement therapy have slower emptying of solids than do men [22, 23, 54]. Whether the GI hypomotility effect of female sex steroids is due to an effect upon gut membranes per se, the anti-aldosterone activity in the case of progesterone or a special role for hormone receptors is not presently known. In favor of a direct progesterone effect is the demonstration that rat antral motility in vitro is significantly inhibited when progesterone is administered in vivo [10].

Calcitonin, used in the treatment of hypercalcemia, causes a pronounced inhibition of GE [61, 62]. The mechanism of delayed GE by calcitonin is unclear. It is unrelated to extracellular calcium concentrations because relatively constant serum levels of calcium and phosphorusare observed throughout the slowed GE during infusion of calcitonin. Likewise, in man as contrasted to in vitro animal models, calcitonin does not decrease gastrin release [62].

2.5 Psychiatric Drugs

Sedative drugs such as the barbiturates, chloral hydrate, hydroxyzine, and paraldehyde can delay GE with the general decrease in GI motility which accompanies drowsiness and sleep. As an example, sedative doses of the barbiturates cause a reduction in tone and motility of the GI tract (including gastric motility) which is believed due to their central depressant action rather than to any direct effects on the tract. Similarly, the anticholinergic activity of certain antihistamines (e. g., diphenhydramine) tricyclic antidepressants, and phenothiazines inhibits gastric motility and delays GE. The tricyclic drug desmethylimipramine has been shown to delay absorption of phenylbutazone in man, and the investigators suggested that this reflects the anticholinergic effect of the drug [20]. Delayed GE by tricyclic antidepressants could however result from both their anticholinergic and norepinephrine enhancing properties. It appears that anxiolytic drugs do not delay GE. A study using oral diazepam showed enhanced gastroduodenal motility and accelerated GE, and another using intramuscular diazepam showed no effect upon GE [109]. Because of the variety of GI motility disorders in which anxiety is believed to play a role, combinations of anticholinergic and anxiolytic drugs are frequently prescribed. The opposing effects of these components upon GE makes prediction of the final effect of any one of these combination drugs difficult.

As an example, the effect of a combination of chlordiazepoxide and clidinium and that of its components alone on GE of a semisolid meal was observed [18]. The combination product increased (antimuscarinic effect) the GE time (mean GE half-time 67 min compared with placebo 55 min), whereas chlordiazepoxide alone (mean GE half-time 55 min), and clidinium alone (59 min) did not do so (Table 5). The data suggest that a synergistic effect by both components contributes to a delay in GE which does not occur with either component alone.

Parenteral lithium acutely inhibits GE in rats; however, lithium had no effect on GE in seven normal human volunteers [25].

2.6 Antipyretics and Nonnarcotic Analgesics

The effects of prostaglandins on GE are complex, with some compounds stimulating and others delaying [83, 107]. Prostaglandin E_1, used intravenously in neonates to maintain patency of the ductus arteriosus, causes delayed GE by induction of antral hyperplasia [89]. However, oral prostaglandin E_1 given to adults in the management of peptic ulcer is not known to effect GE.

The effect of the prostaglandin synthesis inhibitor indomethacin on GE was studied in ten elderly men (aged 69–86, mean age 77) using the radioisotope technique and a Carnation instant breakfast, milk and egg

Table 5. Gastric emptying times (min)

Subject no.	Librax	Clidinium	Chlordiazepoxide	Placebo
1	54	34	31	44
2	80	77	67	83
3	104	70	61	72
4	57	66	62	55
5	69	50	53	58
6	54	65	42	39
7	48	59	40	32
8	104	58	67	66
9	68	66	70	57
10	41	50	61	47
11	70	62	60	65
12	55	54	49	43
Mean $\pm$ SD	67 ± 20.3	59.2 ± 11.3	55.2 ± 12.3	55.1 ± 14.8

Standard error of the difference between two means = 4.05. Significance (P values) for comparisons: Librax > placebo, 0.006 Librax > chlordiazepoxide, 0.007 Librax > clidinium, 0.064 chlordiazepoxide versus placebo, 0.967 clidinium versus placebo, 0.310 clidinium versus chlordiazepoxide, 0.330.

powder meal; and no significant effect was seen (Table 6) [13]. The prostaglandin synthetase inhibitor acetaminophen (paracetamol) is widely used as a systemic antipyretic and analgesic, appearing in more than 200 formulations. The drug has analgesic capability but does not have antiinflammatory or antirheumatic properties, a paradox explained by the differential in sensitivity to the drug by central and peripheral tissue synthetases. A study of gastric emptying following paracetamol ingestion by 11 healthy subjects gave varied results, with three patterns of motility observed in this small series [105].
Interleukin 1-beta is a cytokine isolated from certain cells including lymphocytes and macrophages. It stimulates prostaglandin E_2 synthesis in

Table 6. Gastric emptying times in ten patients (from [13])

Age (years)	Baseline	After placebo, 3 days	After indomethacin, 3 days
69	50	42	42
72	60	ND	64
76	82	64	59
76	43	ND	40
77	35	27	16
78	57	71	78
83	71	68	57
83	ND	78	94
85	99	125	93
86	45	71	57

ND, data not available.

animals and in addition to its gastric cytoprotective action has been shown to delay GE in rats [97].

2.7 Recreational Drugs

Various drugs are consumed in recreational use. These agents include the chemicals in cigarettes, alcoholic beverages, narcotic drugs such as heroin, morphine and its derivatives, cannabis, and the amphetamines. In addition to nicotine, cigarettes contain carbon monoxide, nitrous oxides, and other chemical and physical agents whose separate and cumulative effects upon gastric motility are undefined. The absence of such data may explain why the literature describing changes in gastric motility due to cigarette smoking has been described as "sparse and controversial" [77]. Cigarette smoking accelerated the rate at which the liquid component of a meal leaves the stomach in one report [44] but did not increase liquid-phase GE in another [91]. Smoking high nicotine cigarettes delays solid food GE in normal subjects and patients with active duodenal ulcer. This is believed due to stimulation of duodenogastric reflux and to inhibition of antral motility [47, 84, 85]. Since abstinence from cigarette smoking also has pharmacologic significance (e.g., bioavailability of theophylline), it is of interest that comparison of GE after overnight abstinence and after smoking two cigarettes in 30 min showed no significant difference [91]. Another study found that more rapid GE of a small solid meal induced by cigarettes persisted after 10 h of abstinence [45].

Nicotine is of clinical interest because of its presence in cigarettes, other tobacco products, and snuff because of the phenomenon of nicotine dependence and because nicotine is an approved adjunct to smoking cessation therapies. The introduction of nicotine polacrilex gum as an adjunct to smoking cessation therapy provides a source of nicotine via buccal absorption which is metabolized in a fashion similar to the nicotine in cigarettes, and provides pharmacokinetic data which has a direct application to individuals who use the gum, chew tobacco, or take snuff. A study [14] in ten chronic cigarette smokers who refrained from smoking cigarettes overnight did not show a difference in GE of a semisolid meal when placebo and nicotine gum was chewed after ingestion of the meal. Experimental error due to gum chewing [99] may be avoided in future studies following the increased availability of transdermal nicotine preparations.

Delayed and rapid GE have both been described following ethanol intake. Delayed emptying of liquid and solid meals due to alcohol has been reported in man [4, 59], while other observers have reported accelerated emptying of a liquid meal after acute ethanol administration. Studies using high concentrations of alcohol such as occur in whiskey delay emptying of a standard meal [4], but the lower concentrations found in wine do not affect GE of liquids or solids [75]. GE is delayed in patients with gastroesophageal reflux [71]. Reflux is frequently associated with the esophageal motor dysfunction and lower esophageal sphincter incompetence induced by alcohol. However, the relationship between reflux and GE in the alcoholic population has not been well defined.

Studies using labeled liquid food in lightly anesthetized cats suggest that the delayed GE due to ethanol persists during a 24-h withdrawal period [114]. A study of ten alcoholics who had abstained for the longer period of 3–10 days found no abnormality in the rate of GE at the end of that time [64].

Morphine and other narcotic analgesics increase the tone of the GI smooth muscle, interfere with normal peristalsis, and delay GE [82]. This inhibition of GE by morphine involves drug action via opiate receptors. Naloxone is an opiate receptor antagonist, but 5-mg intravenous boluses does not significantly speed up solid or liquid emptying [74]. Opiate analgesics are considered the major cause of delayed GE seen during the perioperative period [80]. Gastric effects of morphine are supplemented as causes of delayed GE by the powerful duodenal contractions induced by morphine [40]. These effects of narcotic analgesics (and pentazocine) are not reversed by metoclopramide [82]. One would expect diacetylmorphine (heroin) to share these properties, and in one report the mean time to empty 50 % of an ingested solution from the stomach was prolonged from 12 min in controls to more than 130 min after 10 mg heroin administered intramuscularly [79]. The effect of diamorphine on GE does not appear to be chronic, with eight heroin-dependent males exhibiting normal GE of a liquid (glucose solution) meal 20–150 min (mean 61) after their last injection of 10–40 mg (mean 22.5) of the drug [40]. The oral administration of the alkaloid cocaine is followed by peak plasma concentrations within 15 min, suggesting that there is no delay in GE. However, formal studies of GE effects during episodic administration or while tolerance is being developed [1] have not been performed.

The effect of cannabis upon GE is poorly defined, although it has been shown that GE of liquids is unaffected by the intravenous injection of 0.5 and 1 mg delta-9-tetrahydrocannabinol given over a 5-min period [5]. The frequent sideeffects of xerostomia and somnolence suggest a possible delaying effect upon GE when they occur, but this has not been investigated. The use of this drug as an antiemetic agent in oncology may lead to further investigations of its GI effects, which will include measurements of GE [93].

The amphetamines are widely used for their central nervous system stimulating and anorexigenic effects. They are noncatechol sympathomimetic amines with greater central nervous system stimulant activity than epinephrine and other catecholamines. They also have a peripheral action believed to combine release of norepinephrine from adrenergic nerve terminal stores with a direct action on both alpha- and beta-sympathomimetic receptor sites. Fenfluramine is an amphetamine congener which is used as an anorexigenic agent. A study of GE in obese human subjects using a radioisotopic solid meal has shown a significant delay in GE following ingestion of the drug. Fenfluramine had no effect on the gastric emptying of a liquid meal [49, 50].

2.8 Bulking Agents

Echographic studies have shown a correlation between GE and hunger ($p = 0.0007$). When psyllium was added to a standard meal (440 kcal, 600 ml), psyllium slowed GE from the 3rd h while prolonging satiety and delaying hunger [6].

2.9 Antibiotics

Erythromycin, although free of serious adverse reactions, has long been associated with GI side effects, including nausea, vomiting, and diarrhea. Although initial reports suggested that these side effects occur in only 7 %–10 % of subjects receiving oral erythromycin [43], recent studies suggest that up to 51 % of subjects receiving oral erythromycin and 95 % of those receiving intravenous erythromycin experience GI symptoms [65, 94, 106]. In a study of ten subjects given 800 mg erythromycin lactobionate intravenously, eight experienced stomach discomfort, six were nauseated, and one vomited. There was a significant correlation between the severity of symptoms, infusion rate, and plasma erythromycin level [28].

The propensity of erythromycin to produce GI side effects was once ascribed to its antibiotic effect upon the intestinal flora. However, two studies reported in 1984 [57, 92] indicated that erythromycin has a direct effect on GI motility which could be the mechanism whereby GI side effects are induced. Pilot et al. [92] reported the effect of intravenous erythromycin on gastric antral, duodenal, and ileal motor activity in fasted conscious dogs. Intravenous infusion of a subtherapeutic bolus dose of erythromycin (1 mg/kg) stimulated a burst of contractions which originated in the proximal stomach and were propagated to the ileum. Propagation of preceding migratory motor complex (MMC) was abolished and normal fasting activity altered, with continuous irregular activity recorded from stomach to ileum. The higher doses of 7 mg/kg caused an increase in electrical activity at all sites, and all animals vomited. It was concluded that the stimulation of small bowel motility by erythromycin might account for the GI side effects. These results were confirmed by Itoh et al. [57] who also investigated the GI side effects of erythromycin.

The erythromycin-induced contractions in fasted dogs were similar to the naturally occurring MMC and identical to those induced by intravenous infusion of motilin i.e., they all originated in the stomach and were propagated caudally. There was a significant rise of plasma motilin during erythromycin infusion. Subsequently, Peeters and associates [88] showed that motilin accelerates GE in diabetic gastroparesis and hypothesized that erythromycin's effect in man is mediated through motilin receptors. Pentagastrin and feeding inhibited the erythromycin-induced contractions in a similar fashion to motilin, suggesting that erythromycin exerted its effect on small bowel motility through release of endogenous motilin, although the mechanism for this release was obscure. The effect of erythromycin on GI motility was found to be dose dependent: less than $50\,\mu g\ kg^{-1}\ h^{-1}$ failed to stimulate motor activity while doses of $200–400\,\mu g\ kg^{-1}\ h^{-1}$ induced strong contractions which failed to migrate to the proximal jejunum.

Erythromycin has similar effects on antroduodenal motility in man: doses of $1–3\,mg\ kg^{-1}\ h^{-1}$ stimulate MMC-like motor activity [101, 110]. However, plasma motilin does not rise with erythromycin in man, suggesting that erythromycin stimulates MMC activity in man in a different way than it does in dogs.

Otterson and Sarna [86] have reported in more detail the effect of erythromycin on GI motor activity in dog using different doses of oral and intravenous routes. Low doses (1 mg/kg) induced premature MMCs and slowed the migration velocity of MMC. At higher doses, erythromycin did not induce a premature MMC but altered the cycle length of first MMC. At all doses, erythromycin disrupted the MMC in progress. Erythromycin also disrupted the normal electrical control activity of the proximal small bowel and induced what the authors described as "amyogenesis", meaning contractions which occur without the spatial and temporal control of the electrical control activity and are usually disorganized.

Infusion of lipids into the duodenum is known to reduce antral contractility and stimulate localized pyloric contractions, with resulting delayed GE. Intravenous erythromycin overcomes this effect, as shown by a study in 17 normal volunteers whose antral, pyloric, and duodenal motility were measured during small intestinal nutrient infusion with accompanying intravenous erythromycin and intravenous saline [39].

In addition to its effect on antroduodenal motility, erythromycin also exerts effects on other areas of the GI tract, including the lower esophageal sphincter, ileum, colon, gall bladder, and sphincter of Oddi. A detailed description of these actions is beyond the scope of this chapter.

Recent evidence suggests that erythromycin augments GI motility through its action as a motilin receptor agonist [26, 66, 87]. The characteristics of the motor stimulating action of erythromycin on the GI tract are similar to those of motilin. However, the plasma motilin level is increased by erythromycin in dogs but not in man [101, 110]. The action of erythromycin on GI motility appears to be species specific. While erythromycin causes a dose-dependent contraction of isolated rabbit's duodenal (to a lesser extent of gastric, ileal, and colonic) muscle strips, the rat and guinea pig smooth muscle strips do not contract in response to erythromycin [87]. Motilin shows a similar species specificity and activity profile. The erythromycin-induced smooth muscle contractions in the rabbit were not inhibited by atropine, hexamethonium, naloxone, diphenhydramine, methysergide, procaine, trypsin, indomethacin, or sodium nitroprusside but were blocked by nifedipine, indicating that the action of erythromycin is calcium dependent [3]. The action of erythromycin on GI motility does not appear to be related to its antibacterial activity because the derivative of erythromycin (EM-536) with no antibacterial activity also has motilinlike activity, in fact 2890 times more

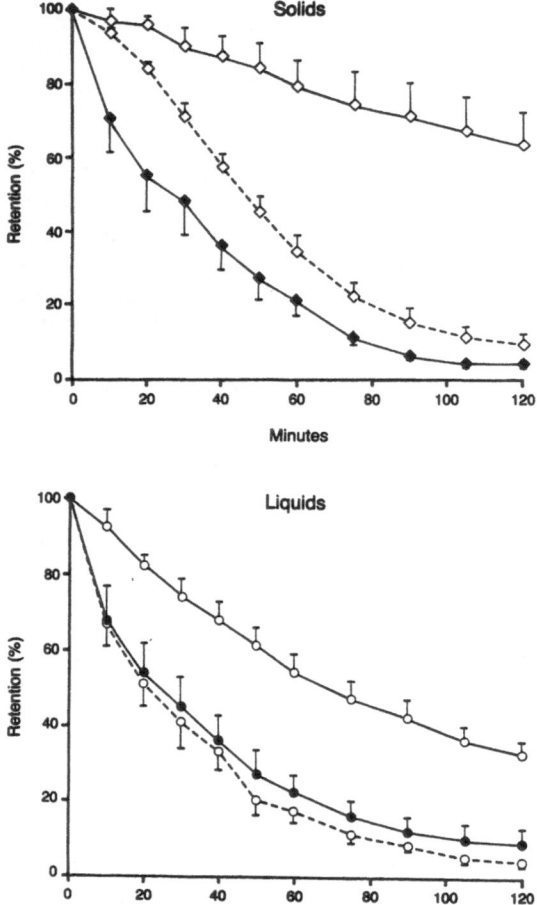

Fig. 4. Effect of erythromycin on GE time (GET). *Above,* GET of solid meal: *upper curve,* ten diabetic patients receiving intravenous placebo showing delayed GET; *lower curve,* ten diabetic patients receiving a single intravenous dose of 200 mg erythromycin showing accelerated GET; *middle curve,* GET in ten control healthy subjects. *Below,* GET of liquid meal: *upper curve,* ten diabetic patients receiving placebo showing delayed GET; *middle curve,* ten diabetic patients receiving a single intravenous dose of 200 mg erythromycin showing improvement in GET; *lower curve,* GET in ten control healthy subjects. (Reproduced with permission from [58])

potent than erythromycin itself. Thus, it appears that erythromycin and its analogues stimulate GI contraction by acting directly on the motilin receptor on smooth muscle via a calcium dependent system. Neural mechanisms do not appear to play a role.

There also appears to be a structure-activity relationship on the action of erythromycin on GI motility. Erythromycin belongs to a chemical group called macrolides (a giant lactone nucleus consisting of many carbon atoms), which fall into two categories depending on the number of carbon atoms in the lactone ring – 14 or 16. Oleandomycin, a 14-membered macrolide like erythromycin, was found to stimulate antral motor activity in the dog in a similar fashion to erythromycin, but it is 20 times less potent than erythromycin. On the other hand, the 16-membered macrolides (including josamycin, spiramycin, leukomycin, acetylspiramycin, and tylosin) have no GI contractile activity, and these compounds are not associated with side effects in clinical use [12]. Figure 4 shows the effect of erythromycin on gastric emptying.

3 Discussion

The rate of GE influences the rate at which drugs are absorbed. Most pathological states and secondary drug effects which alter GE do so by delaying GE. At present, the dumping syndrome is the only disorder characterized by too-rapid emptying in which treatment is aimed specifically at the GE rate. The stomach is not an important site of drug absorption, so that for any drug where a rapid therapeutic effect is required, delayed GE impedes success. Delayed GE may result in subtherapeutic drug concentrations in the tissues despite intake of an appropriate oral dose in drugs such as procainamide or penicillin whose short biological half-life makes them susceptible to intragastric degradation [79]. Delayed GE which is not recognized preoperatively has potential for increased vomiting and aspiration during the perioperative period. The availability of gastrokinetic agents has greatly increased the clinical value of GE data, but it must be emphasized that these data cannot be extrapolated to direct predictions about the systemic availability of an oral agent. An example is provided by levodopa, a drug which is sensitive to metabolism by an enzyme (dopa decarboxylase) with high activity in the gastric mucosa. As a result one would expect the slower GE found in elderly parkinsonian and nonparkinsonian patients to reduce systemic availability of the drug in the elderly. Instead, it has been shown that the increased residence time of levodopa in the stomach of the elderly is associated with enhanced systemic availability of the drug [33], apparently explained by an age-related decrease in the activity of dopa decarboxylase in the gastric mucosa. Another caveat is the factor introduced by synergistic or antagonistic effects of simultaneously administered drugs upon GE, as exemplified by an association of clidinium + chlordiazepoxide [18].

The administration of prokinetic drugs for delayed GE requires careful monitoring for an accurate appraisal of their clinical value. Yet drugs such as chlorpromazine which have prominent central actions could ameliorate nausea and vomiting symptomatology without accelerating GE [36]. In spite of these difficulties, continued study of drug effects upon GE is clearly indicated as part of the endeavor to put therapeutics on an ever more rational and predictable basis.

4 Conclusion

The bioavailability of orally administered medication may be significantly altered by an effect of that medication or other simultaneously administered drugs upon GE. New techniques for measuring GE rates and the advent of new prokinetic agents has increased our understanding of the factors which effect GE and our ability to intervene therapeutically when GE rates are abnormal.

References

1. Ambre, JJ, Belknap, SM, Nelson, J, Ruo, TI, Shin, SG, Atkinson, AJ JR (1988) Acute tolerance to cocaine in humans. Clin Pharmacol Ther 44: 1–8
2. Amidon, GL, DeBrinkat, GA, Najib, N (1991) Effects of gravity on gastric emptying, intestinal transit, and drug absorption. J Clin Pharmacol 31: 968–973
3. Bani, M, Cosiovich, B, Fiorentini, F, Sfriso, L, Guarneri, L (1988) Analysis of the motor stimulating effect of erythromycin on gastrointestinal tract in vitro. Hepatogastroenterology 35: 196
4. Barboriak, JJ, Meade, RC (1970) Effect of alcohol on gastric emptying in man. Am J Clin Nutr 23: 1151–1153
5. Bateman, DN (1983) Delta-9-tetrahydrocannabinol and gastric emptying. Br J Clin Pharmac 15: 749–751
6. Bergmann, JF, Chassany, O, Caulin, C, Segrestaa, JM (1992) Correlation between echographic gastric emptying and appetite; influence of psyllium. Gastroenterology 102: A 425
7. Berkowitz, DM, McCallum, RW (1980) Interaction of levodopa and metoclopramide on gastric emptying. Clin Pharmacol Ther 27: 414–420
8. Blackwell, JN, Holt, S, Heading, RC (1981) Effect of nifedipine on esophageal motility and gastric emptying. Digestion 21: 50–56
9. Bromster, D, Carlberger, G, Lundh, G, Moller, J, Rosen, A (1969) The effect of some oral anticholinergics on gastric emptying, pH and osmolarity in man. Scand J Gastroenterol 4: 192–195
10. Bruce, LA, Behsudi, FZ (1979) Progesterone effects on three regional gastrointestinal tissues. Life Sci 25: 729–734
11. Bruley, des Varannes, S, Parys, V, Chayvialle, JA, Gaimiche, JP (1992) In humans, erythromycin (EM) increases proximal gastric tone without endogenous motilin release. Gastroenterology 102: A 432
12. Catnach, SM, Fairclough, PD (1992) Erythromycin and the gut. Gut 33: 397–401

13. Chaudhuri, TK, Fink, S (1984) Lack of effect of indomethacin on gastric emptying in old men. J Amer Geriatrics Society 32: 19–20
14. Chaudhuri, TK, Fink, S (1988) The effect of nicotine upon gastric emptying. Clin Res 36: 394 A (abstract)
15. Chaudhuri, TK, Fink, S (1989) Nifedipine and gastric emptying. Dig Dis Sci 34: 157–158
16. Chaudhuri, TK, Fink, S, Goetsch, RA (1985) Correlation of cardiovascular and gastric effects of nifedipine. Circulation 72: III-275 (abstract)
17. Chaudhuri, TK, Fink, S, Goetsch, RA (1986) Effect of nifedipine on gastric emptying. J Nucl Med 27: 905 (abstract)
18. Chaudhuri, TK, Hudgins, MH (1982) Effect of Librium, Quarzan and Librax on gastric emptying. J Nucl Med 23: P 21
18a. Chernish, SM, Brunelle, RR, Rosenak, DB, Ahmadzai, S (1978) Comparison of the effects of glucagon and atropine sulfate on gastric emptying. Am J Gastroenterol 70: 581–586
19. Clark, JM, Seager, SJ (1983) Gastric emptying following premedication with glycopyrrolate or atropine. Br J Anaesth 55: 1195–1199
20. Consolo, S, Morselli, PL, Zaccala, M, Garattini, S (1970) Delayed absorption of phenylbutazone caused by desmethylimipramine in humans. Eur J Pharmacol 10: 239–242
21. Corinaldesi, R, Scarpignato, C, Galassi, A, Stanghellini, V, Calamelli, R, Bertaccini, G, Barbara, L (1984) Effect of ranitidine and cimetidine on gastric emptying of a mixed meal in man. International J Clin Pharmacology, Therapy and Toxicology 22: 498–501
22. Datz, FL, Christian, PE, Moore, JG (1986) Sex-related differences in gastric emptying. J Nucl Med 27: 904 (abstract)
23. Datz, FL, Christian, PE, Moore JG.(1987 a) Differences in gastric emptying rates between menstruating and postmenopausal women. J Nucl Med 28: 604 (abstract)
24. Datz, FL, Christian, PE, Moore, JG (1987 b) Gender-related differences in gastric emptying. J Nucl Med 28: 1204–1207
25. DeMarkles, MP, Sjogren, R, Peller, P, Maydonovitch, C, Wong, RKH (1992) Effect of lithium carbonate on gastric emptying, gastric electrophysiology, GI hormones in humans. Gastroenterology 102: A 441
26. Depoortere, I, Peeters, TL, Matthijs, G, Vantrappen, G (1988) Macrolides antibiotics are motilin receptor agonists. Hepatogastroenterology 35: 198
27. Di Somma, C, Arnulfo, C, Mortola, G et al. (1986) Effects of pirenzepine and atropine on gastroduodenal motor patterns in duodenal ulcer patients. Scand J Gastroenterol 21: 1046–1050
28. Downey, KM, Chaput de Saintonge, DM (1986) Gastrointestinal side effects after intravenous erythromycin lactobionate. Br J Clin Pharmacol 21: 295–299
29. Dubois, A, Castell, DO (1986) Histamine H2-receptor involvement in the regulation of gastric emptying. Am J Physiol 250 (Gastrointest Liver Physiol 13): G 244-247
30. Dubois, A, Castell, DO (1987) Reply to Scarpignato "Are H2-receptors involved in the physiological regulation of gastric emptying?" Am J Physiol 252: G 720
31. Dubois, A, Nompleggi, D, Myers, L, Castell, DO (1978) Histamine H2 receptor stimulation increases gastric emptying. Gastroenterology 74: 1028
32. Ettman, IK, Bonchillon CD, Halford, HH (1957) Gastrointestinal roentgen findings due to untoward effects of hexamethonium. Radiology 68: 673–678
33. Evans, MA, Broe, GA, Triggs, EJ, Cheung, M, Creasey, H, Paull, PD (1981) Gastric emptying rate and the systemic availability of levodopa in the elderly parkinsonian patient. Neurology 31: 1288–1294
34. Fink, S, Chaudhuri, TK (1985) Gastric side effect of nifedipine. Amer J Gastroenterology 80: 839 (abstract)

35. Fink, S, Friedman, G (1960) The differential effect of drugs upon the proximal and distal colon of man. Am J Med 28: 534–538

36. Fink, S, Winslow, WA (1955) Anti-emetic effect of chlorpromazine in cancer patients. Gastroenterology 28: 731–734

37. Fraser, R, Horowitz, M, Maddox, A, Harding, P, Chatterton, B, Dent, J (1990) Hyperglycaemia slows gastric emptying in type 1 (insulin-dependent) diabetes mellitus. Diabetologia 33: 675–680

38. Fraser, R, Fuller, J, Horowitz, M, Dent, J (1991) Effect of insulin-induced hypoglycaemia on antral, pyloric and dodenal motility in fasting subjects. Clin Sci 81: 281–285

39. Fraser, R, Shearer, T, Fuller, J, Horowitz, M, Dent, J (1992) Intravenous erythromycin overcomes small intestinal feedback on antral, pyloric and duodenal motility. Gastroenterology 103: 114–119

40. Ghodse, AH, Reed, JL (1984) Gastric emptying, glucose tolerance and associated hormonal changes in heroin addiction. Psychological Medicine 14: 521–525

41. Goetsch, RA, Fink, S, Chaudhuri, TK (1986) Effect of nifedipine on gastric emptying. Military Medicine 151: 438–439

42. Goodall, P (1970) The effect of hexamethonium and atropine on gastric emptying of hyperosmolar glucose solution. Brit J Surg 57: 857

43. Griffith, RS, Black, HR (1970) Erythromycin. Med Clin N Amer 54: 1199–1215

44. Grimes, DS, Goddard, J (1978) Effect of cigarette smoking on gastric emptying. Br Med J 2: 460–461

45. Hanson, M, Lilja, B (1987) Gastric emptying in smokers. Scand J Gastroenterol 22: 1102–1104

46. Harasawa, A, Kikuchi, K, Senoue, I, Nomiyama, T, Miwa, T (1982) Gastric emptying in patients with gastric ulcers. Effects of oral and intramuscular administration of anticholinergic drug. Tokai J Exp Clin Med 7: 551–559

47. Harrison, A, Ippolit, A (1979) Effect of smoking on gastric emptying. Gastroenterology 76: 1152

48. Health, and Public Policy Committee, American College of Physicians (1986) Methods for stopping cigarette smoking. Ann Intern Med 105: 281–291

49. Horowitz, M (1987) Fenfluramine and gastric emptying. Am J Physiol 252: R 433

50. Horowitz, M, Collins, PJ, Tuckwell, V, Vernon-Roberts, J, Shearman, DJC (1985) Fenfluramine delays gastric emptying of solid food. Br J Clin Pharmac 19: 849–851

51. Hunt, JN, Pathak, JD (1960) The osmotic effects of some simple molecules and ions on gastric emptying. J Physiol 154: 254–269

52. Hurwitz, A, Robinson, R, Christie, J, Herrin, W (1979) Delayed gastric emptying after anticholinergic drugs. Clin Pharmac Therap 25: 230

53. Hutson, WR, Roehrkasse, R, Kaslewicz, F, Stoney, B, Wald, A (1987) Influence of sex and weight on gastric emptying and antral motility. Gastroenterology 92: 1443 (abstract)

54. Hutson, WR, Roehrkasse, R, Wald, A (1989) Influence of gender and menopause on gastric emptying and motility. Gastroenterology 96: 11–17

55. Hutson, WR, Wald, A (1987) Sex and menopausal status of subjects in gastric emptying studies. J Nucl Med 28: 1926–1927 (letter to the editor)

56. Imbimbo, BP, Gardino, L, Palmas, F, Frascio, M, Canepa, G, Scarpignato, C (1990) Different effects of atropine and cimetropium bromide on gastric emptying of liquids and antroduodenal motor activity in man. Hepatogastroenterology 37: 242–246

57. Itoh, Z, Nakaya, M, Suzuki, T, Arai, H, Wakabayashi, K (1984) Erythromycin mimics exogenous motilin in gastrointestinal contractile activity in the dog. Am J Physiol 247: G 688–694

58. Janssens, J, Peeters, TL, Vantrappen, G, Tack, J, Urbain, JL, DeRoo, M, Muls, E, Bouillon, R (1990) Improvement of gastric emptying in diabetic gastroparesis by erythromycin: preliminary studies. NEJM 322: 1028–1031
59. Jian, R, Cortot, A, Ducrot, F, Jobin, G, Chayvialle, JA, Modigliani, R (1986) Effect of ethanol ingestion on postprandial gastric emptying and secretion, biliopancreatic secretions, and duodenal absorption in man. Dig Dis Sci 31: 604–614
60. Johannesson, N, Andersson, K-E, Joelsson, B, Persson, CGA (1985) Relaxation of lower esophageal sphincter and stimulation of gastric secretion and diuresis by antiasthmatic xanthines. Am Rev Respir Dis 131: 26–30
61. Jonderko, G, Golab, T, Jonderko, K (1987) Calcitonin suppresses gastric emptying of a radiolabeled solid meal in humans. Brit J Clin Pharmac 24: 103–105
62. Jonderko, K, Jonderko, G, Golab, T (1990) Effect of calcitonin on gastric emptying and on serum insulin and gastrin concentrations after ingestion of a mixed solid-liquid meal in humans. J Clin Gastroenterol 12: 22–28
63. Kawamoto, H, Yamamura, HY, Tatsuta M, Okuda, S (1985) Effect of glucagon on gastric motility examined by the acetaminophen absorption method and the endoscopic procedure. Arzneim Forsch/Drug Res 35: 1475–1477
64. Keshavarzian, A, Iber, FL, Greer, P, Wobbleton, J (1986) Gastric emptying of solid meal in male chronic alcoholics. Alcohol: Clin Exp Res 10: 432–435
65. Klika, LJ, Goodman, JM (1982) Gastrointestinal tract symptoms from intravenously administered erythromycin. JAMA 248: 1309
66. Kondo, Y, Torii, K, Itoh, Z, Omura, S (1988) Erythromycin and its derivatives with motilin-like biological activities inhibit the specific binding of I-125-motilin to duodenal muscle. Biochem Biophys Res Commun 150: 877–882
67. Lin, HC, Moller, NA, Wolinsky, MM, Kim, BH, Doty, JE, Meyer, JH (1992) Sustained slowing effect of lentils on gastric emptying of solids in humans and dogs. Gastroenterology 102: 787–792
68. Logan, RFA, Forrest, JAH, McLoughlin, GP, Lidgard, G, Heading, RC (1978) Effect of cimetidine on serum gastrin and gastric emptying in man. Digestion 18: 220-226
69. MacGregor, IL, Gueller, R, Watts, H, Meyer, J (1976) The effects of acute hyperglycaemia on gastric emptying in man. Gastroenterology 70: 190–196
70. Marano, AR, Caride, VJ, Prokop, EK, Troncale, FJ, McCallum, RW (1985) Effect of sucralfate and an aluminum hydroxide gel on gastric emptying of solids and liquids. Clin Pharmacol Ther 37: 629–632
71. McCallum, RW, Fink, SM, Lerner, E, Berkowitz, DM (1983) Effects of metoclopramide and bethanechol on delayed gastric emptying present in gastroesophageal reflux patients. Gastroenterology 84: 1573–1577
72. McEvoy, GK (ed) (1991) Antimuscarinics/antispasmodics. In: American Hospital Formulary Service. Bethesda, Md: American Society of Hospital Pharmacists 645–670
73. McEvoy, GK (ed) (1986) Miscellaneous autonomic drugs. In: American Hospital Formulary Service. Bethesda, Md: American Society of Hospital Pharmacists 657–662
74. Mittal, RK, Frank, EB, Lange, RC, McCallum, RW (1986) Effects of morphine and naloxone on esophageal motility and gastric emptying in man. Dig Dis Sci 31: 936–942
75. Moore, JG, Christian, PE, Datz, FL (1981) Effect of wine on gastric emptying in humans. Gastroenterology 81: 1072–1075
76. Moore, JG, Tweedy, C, Christian, PE, Datz, FL (1983) Effect of age on gastric emptying of liquid-solid meals in man. Dig Dis Sci 28: 340–344
77. Muller-Lissner, SA (1986) Bile reflux is increased in cigarette smokers. Gastroenterology 90: 1205–1209
78. Muller-Lissner, SA, Fraas, C, Hartl, A (1986) Cisapride offsets dopamine-induced slowing of fasting gastric emptying. Dig Dis Sci 31: 807–810

79. Nimmo, WS (1976) Drugs, diseases, and altered gastric emptying. Clin Pharmacokinetics 1: 189–203
80. Nimmo, WS (1984) Effect of anaesthesia on gastric motility and emptying. Br J Anaesth 56: 29–36
81. Nimmo, J, Heading, RC, Tothill, P, Prescott, LF (1973) Pharmacological modification of gastric emptying: effects of propantheline and metoclopramide on paracetamol absorption. Br Med J 1: 587–589
82. Nimmo, WS, Heading, RC, Wilson, J, Tothill, P, Prescott, LF (1975) Inhibition of gastric emptying and drug absorption by narcotic analgesics. Brit J Clin Pharmacol 2: 509–513
83. Nompleggi, D, Myers, L, Castell, DO, Dubois, A (1980) Effect of a prostaglandin E2 analog on gastric emptying and secretion in rhesus monkeys. J Pharmacol Exp Ther 212: 491–495
84. Nowak, A, Jonderko, K, Kaczor, R, Nowak, S, Skrzypek, D (1987a) Cigarette smoking delays gastric emptying of a radiolabelled solid food in healthy smokers. Scand J Gastroenterol 22: 54–58
85. Nowak, A, Jonderko, K, Kaczor, R, Nowak, S, Skrzypek, D (1987b) Effect of cigarette smoking on gastric emptying in patients with an active duodenal ulcer. Scand J Gastroenterol 22: 1105–1108
86. Otterson, MF, Sarna, SK (1990) Gastrointestinal motor effects of erythromycin. Amer J Physiol 259: G 355–363
87. Peeters, TL, Matthija, G, Depoortere, I, Cachet, T, Hoogmartens, J, Vantrappen, G (1989) Erythromycin is a motilin receptor agonist. Am J Physiol 257: G 470–474
88. Peeters, TL, Muls, E, Janssens, J, Urbain, J-L, Bex, M, Van Cutsem, E, Depoortere, I, DeRoo, M, Vantrappen, G, Bouillon, R (1992) Effect of motilin on gastric emptying in patients with diabetic gastroparesis. Gastroenterology 102: 97–101
89. Peled, N, Dagan, O, Babyn, P, Silver, MM, Barker, G, Hellmann, J, Scolnik, D, Koren, G (1992) Gastric-outlet obstruction induced by prostaglandin therapy in neonates. NEJM 327: 505–510
90. Petersen, JM, Caride, VJ, Prokop, EK, Troncale, FJ, McCallum, RW (1985) Sucralfate delays gastric emptying of solid and liquid components of a meal in duodenal ulcer patients. Proc 50th Annual Scientific Meeting of the American College of Gastroenterology, Miami, Fla, P-124
91. Petring, OU, Adelhoj, B, Ibsen, M, Brynnum, J, Poulsen, HE (1985) Abstaining from cigarette smoking has no major effect on gastric emptying in habitual smokers. Br J Anaesth 57: 1104–1106
92. Pilot, MA, Ritchie, HD, Thompson, H, Zara, GP (1984) Alterations in gastrointestinal motility associated with erythromycin. Br J Pharmacol 81: 168 P (abstract)
93. Poster, DS, Penta, JS, Bruno, S, Macdonald, JS (1981) Delta-9-tetrahydrocannabinol in clinical oncology. JAMA 245: 2047–2051
94. Putzi, R, Blaser, J, Luthy, R, Wehrli, R, Siegenthaler, W (1983) Side effects due to the intravenous infusion of erythromycin. Infection 11: 161–163
95. Rashid, MU, Bateman, DN (1990) Effect of intravenous atropine on gastric emptying, paracetamol absorption, salivary flow and heart rate in young and fit elderly volunteers. Br J Clin Pharmac 30: 25–34
96. Rees, MR, Clark, RA, Holdsworth, CD (1980) The effect of beta-adrenoceptor agonists and antagonists on gastric emptying in man. Br J Clin Pharmacol 10: 551–554
97. Robert, A, Olafsson, AS, Lancaster, C, Zhang, W (1991) Interleukin-1 is cytoprotective, antisecretory, stimulates PGE2 synthesis by the stomach, and retards gastric emptying. Life Sci 48: 123–134
98. Roehrkasse, R, Kaslewicz, F, Stoney, B, Wald, A (1986) Sex differences in gastric emptying and antral motility. Clin Res 34: 953 (abstract)

99. Rose, JE, Herskovic, JE, Trilling, Y, Jarvik, ME (1985) Transdermal nicotine reduces cigarette craving and nicotine preference. Clin Pharmacol Ther 38: 450–455

100. Santander, R, Mena, I, Gramisu, M, Valenzuela, JE (1988) Effect of nifedipine on gastric emptying and gastrointestinal motility in man. Dig Dis Sc 33: 535–538

101. Sarna, SK, Soergel, KH, Koch, TR, Stone, JE, Wood, CM, Ryan, RP, Cavanaugh, JH, Nellans, HN, Lee, MB (1989) Effects of erythromycin on human gastrointestinal motor activity in the fed and fasted states. Gastroenterology 96: A 440

102. Scarpignato, C, Bertaccini, G (1982) Different effects of cimetidine and ranitidine on gastric emptying in rats and man. Agents and Actions 12: 172–173

103. Scarpignato, C, Heading, RC (1987) Are H2-receptors involved in the physiological regulation of gastric emptying? Am J Physiol 252: G 719–720

104. Scarpignato, C, Bertaccini, G, Zimbaro, G, Vitulo, F (1982) Ranitidine delays gastric emptying of solids in man. Br J Clin Pharmacol 13: 252–253

105. Schurizek, BA, Kraglund, K, Andreasen, F, Vinter-Jensen, L, Juhl, B (1989) Antroduodenal motility and gastric emptying: Gastroduodenal motility and pH following ingestion of paracetamol. Aliment-Pharmacol-Ther 3: 93–101

106. Shanson, DC, Akash, S, Harris, M, Tadayon, M (1985) Erythromycin stearate 1.5 g for the oral prophylaxis of streptococcal bacteremia in patients undergoing dental extraction: efficacy and tolerance. J Antimicrob Chemother 15: 183–190

107. Shea-Donohue, PT, Myers, L, Castell, DO, Dubois, A (1980) Effect of prostacyclin on gastric emptying and secretion in rhesus monkeys. Gastroenterology 74: 1476–1479

108. Steinheber, FU (1985) Ageing and the stomach. Clin Gastroenterol 14: 657–688

109. Todd, JG, Nimmo, WS (1983) Effect of premedication on drug absorption and gastric emptying. Br J Anaesth 55: 1189–1193

110. Tomomasa, T, Kuroume, T, Arai, H, Wakabayashi, K, Itoh, Z (1986) Erythromycin induces migrating motor complex in human gastrointestinal tract. Dig Dis Sci 31: 157–161

111. Traube, M, Lange, RC, MacAllister, RG, McCallum, RW (1985) Effect of nifedipine on gastric emptying in normal subjects. Dig Dis Sc 30: 710–712

112. Tsutsumi, K, Nakashima, H, Kotegawa, T, Nakano, S (1992) Influence of food on the absorption of beta-methyldigoxin. J Clin Pharmacol 32: 157–162

113. Wald, A, Van Thiel, DH, Hoechstetter, L, Gavaler, JS, Egler, KM, Verm, R, Scott, L, Lester, R (1981) Gastrointestinal transit: the effect of the menstrual cycle. Gastroenterology 80: 1497–1500

114. Willson, CA, Bushnell, D, Keshavarazian (1990) The effect of acute and chronic ethanol administration on gastric emptying in cats. Dig Dis Sci 35: 444–448

115. Ziment, I, Au, JP (1986) Ancholinergic agents. Clinics in chest medicine 7: 355–366

Intestinal Damage by Anti-inflammatory Agents

A. Macpherson and I. Bjarnason

Departments of Clinical Biochemistry and Medicine, King's College School of Medicine and Dentistry, London SE5 9PJ, UK.

1 Introduction: Extent of Intestinal Problems with NSAIDs

Non steroidal anti-inflammatory drugs (NSAIDs) are one of the most successful classes of therapeutic agents ever marketed. Hence their adverse effects on the gastrointestinal (GI) tract have become the commonest and most important cause of medically induced iatrogenic GI disease. Unfortunately, the medical community has been lulled into a misunderstanding of the GI site that most commonly suffers complications in patients on NSAIDs. To a large extent this is the consequence of the 'intestinal myopia' which results from the widespread availability of upper GI endoscopes, which rarely progress further than the second part of the duodenum. The ease with which gastroduodenal ulceration can be visualised is emphasised by the dramatic consequences of haemorrhage from a bleeding ulcer. In itself this is certainly a most significant clinical problem. It has been estimated that for every 500–800 prescriptions of NSAIDs, one patient experiences catastrophic GI complications in the shape of haemorrhage or perforation from a peptic ulcer (totalling 30,000–40,000 patients annually in the United Kingdom, and this results in a 10% mortality risk [3, 6, 33, 34, 38, 71]. However, these factors have concealed the fact that the small intestine is the commonest site of NSAID toxicity, resulting in considerable morbidity (and mortality) in chronic users of the drugs.

In this review we outline the techniques used to define small intestinal NSAID enteropathy, and show the extent of the problem and its potential complications in patients on long-term NSAIDs. To give a balanced view of the overall problems of NSAID GI toxicity, we also briefly cover the damage and complications that arise in the gastroduodenal mucosa and in the colon.

2 Small Intestinal NSAID Damage

2.1 Methods of Studying the Effect of NSAIDs on the Small Intestine

A valuable way to identify and quantitate intestinal inflammation caused by NSAIDs is to use the method of ^{111}In labelling of autologous leucocytes. Briefly, a venous blood sample is taken, and the white cell fraction is separated. The neutrophils are labelled *in vitro* with ^{111}In, using tropolone as an ionophore, and reinjected back into the patient. The site of intestinal inflammation can be identified using abdominal scintigrams, and its severity is quantitated by collecting the stool samples from the patient over 4 days; the radioactivity recovered in these stool samples (as percentage of the injected dose) is defined by radioactive counting.

The rationale for the ^{111}In white cell method is that neutrophils maintain their function to migrate into tissue in response to specific neutrophil chemoattractants, and having dealt with the chemoattractant they pass between the epithelial cells in the inflamed intestine [49, 64–66, 68, 82, 83] into the GI lumen. Consequently, the scintigrams show the site at which neutrophils pass through the intestinal mucosa, and once in the lumen the radioactive marker passed in the stools, giving an accurate quantitative measure of the amount of inflammation.

A more sophisticated version of the indium scan can be used to define intestinal bleeding at the same time as the inflammation. This involves separating red cells from the sample of venous blood and labelling them with ^{51}Cr [21]. The sample is then reinjected into the patient at the same time as the autologous leucocytes [10]. The radiolabel is passed into the lumen only if there is intestinal blood loss, and this can be quantitated by comparing the radioactivity of blood (usually 4 ml) from the previous day with the ^{51}Cr activity of stool. As the ^{111}In activity is many orders of magnitude greater than ^{51}Cr and ^{111}In has a much shorter half-life than ^{51}Cr (36 h and 28 days, respectively), ^{111}In activity can be assessed immediately at the end of the faecal collection without interference from ^{51}Cr, and when the ^{111}In has been allowed to decay for a month the ^{51}Cr counts can be obtained.

Many clinicians find themselves with a credibility barrier when faced with the results of investigations depending on radiochemical labelling, particularly as in this case where the samples actually being counted consist of faecal material! For those in whom unfamiliarity or scepticism transposes the Department of Nuclear Medicine into the Department of Unclear Medicine, it is fortunate that there is visible confirmation of the small intestinal abnormalities caused by NSAIDs. This comes from surgical resection specimens, post-mortem pathological material and endoscopy [1, 11, 46, 50, 51]. A new development in endoscopic instrumentation has resulted in production of a thin, flexible enteroscope capable of visualising the entire small intestine. This is passed transnasally and manoevered into the duodenum, when a balloon at the tip of the instrument is inflated, and the length of the enteroscope is gradually introduced as peristalsis carries the tip progressively distally through the small bowel. An excellent view of the mucosa is obtained as the instrument is withdrawn.

2.2 NSAID Enteropathy

2.2.1 Characterisation

The ^{111}In leucocyte method shows no abnormality in patients with rheumatoid or osteoarthritis who have not been treated with NSAIDs, indicating that there is no background intestinal inflammation caused by these diseases themselves [8, 9, 61, 67]. In contrast, in 65 %–70 % of patients who have been treated with NSAIDs for over 6 months there is increased faecal ^{111}In excretion showing intestinal inflammation, and in most of these patients abdominal scintigraphy can identify the inflammatory site as the small intestine.

This largely asymptomatic NSAID enteropathy found in the majority of long-term NSAID users consists of low-grade inflammation, which is of a severity similar to that found in quiescent inflammatory bowel disease, and an order of magnitude less than active ulcerative colitis or Crohn's disease [9]. The actual NSAID prescribed makes no significant difference to the inflammation, either in its severity or its location. One important exception to this is aspirin; this appears rarely to cause small intestinal inflammation, although it is well known to damage the gastroduodenal mucosa.

The NSAID-induced small intestinal inflammation is reversible after discontinuing the drug, albeit slowly, taking up to 18 months to resolve.

Recently the introduction of enteroscopy has allowed direct endoscopic visualisation of NSAID enteropathy [1, 50, 51]. In chronic NSAID users, submucosal haemorrhages and overt mucosal ulcers have been documented in the middle of the small bowel, confirming that in humans (as in experimental animals) the small intestine is the principal site of GI NSAID toxicity.

2.2.2 Complications

Since NSAID enteropathy is largely clinically occult, its significance lies in the complications that may result from the condition. These include GI bleeding and protein loss, which are important iatrogenic causes of morbidity in patients with joint disease on NSAID treatment. Because the enteropathy is not obvious, it is easy to confuse these abnormalities with activity of the underlying disease [17, 36, 78]. Moreover, in the face of anaemia many patients require workup to exclude an occult gastroduodenal ulcer or a neoplasm, and in the past clinicians have been puzzled by the low diagnostic yield from upper GI endoscopy and colonoscopy [4, 5, 8]

2.2.2.1 GI Bleeding. Whilst many patients with rheumatoid arthritis (on NSAIDs) have anaemia of chronic disease, over half those that are anaemic develop iron deficiency, and a few patients develop a pure iron-deficiency picture [17, 36, 78]. The standard workup by upper GI endoscopy almost invariably excludes significant gastroduodenal ulceration that can be blamed for the problem [4, 5, 8]. Dual labelling of leucocytes with ^{111}In and erythrocytes with ^{51}Cr and ^{99m}Tc allows the simultaneous estimation and localisation of GI blood loss and inflammatory enteropathy in NSAID-treated patients, respectively [10]. This shows that (a) those patients with small intestinal inflammation as a result of NSAID treatment have mild chronic blood loss (2–10 ml/day), and (b) the blood loss occurs at the same site as the inflammation, that is, the mid small intestine. There is a further interesting point to emerge from these studies; when patients on NSAIDs have mild abnormalities in the gastroduodenal mucosa because of NSAID treatment such as erosions or submucosal haemorrhages (defined in the studies by concurrent endoscopy), the ^{99m}Tc scans demonstrate that these are **not** the main source of the blood loss which is coming from the small intestinal enteropathy. Of course, the catastrophic GI haemorrhage associated with a bleeding deep chronic peptic ulcer is a quite different circumstance. Unfortunately, it is not possible to predict those patients who will experience dramatic and life-treatening GI haemorrhage from NSAID-associated gastroduodenal ulceration, nor is it possible to exclude an unrelated cause of GI blood loss (such as colonic polyposis or carcinomatosis) without investigation. Undoubtedly the endoscopic workup for iron-deficiency anaemia with upper GI endoscopy and colonoscopy poses considerable demands on resources; whilst this cannot be avoided unless an effective treatment of NSAID enteropathy is developed to eliminate the cause of the problem, it is important to be aware of the concurrent small intestinal bleeding to avoid unnecessarily repeated negative investigations.

2.2.2.2 Protein Loss. Approximately 10 % of hospitalised patients with rheumatoid arthritis have hypoalbuminaemia. In the past this has been attributed to reduced hepatic protein synthesis or intestinal amyloidosis, although there was little concrete evidence for this. It has been shown that NSAID enteropathy may be associated with protein-losing enteropathy by simultaneously labelling leucocytes with ^{111}In and albumin with ^{51}Cr [10]. Once the stools have been collected and the counts from each isotope established, it is apparent that intestinal protein loss accompanies the inflammatory NSAID enteropathy. That this can be a most significant problem is shown by one patient who was studied with hypoalbuminaemia and the intestinal loss of over 300 ml plasma/day. In such cases the hypoalbuminaemia responds to withdrawing NSAID treatment.

2.2.2.3 Diaphragm (Bjarnason's) Disease. One of the most serendipitous complications of NSAID enteropathy is the finding of diaphragmatic strictures of the small intestine [10, 39, 40, 42, 46, 74, 77]. This is a very rare complication, but pathognomic of NSAID damage. Unlike the strictures caused by inflammatory bowel (Crohn's) disease, intestinal lymphoma or excessive potassium supplementation where there is distortion of the lumen, NSAID diaphragms are multiple thin septate strictures in the middle small bowel which can be easily missed on barium follow-through examinations. The patients may be symptomatic with subacute obstruction, but even this may be difficult to differentiate from chronic dyspepsia. It is likely that the diaphragms are most easily diagnosed using enteroscopy, although the experience with this at present is limited.

2.2.3 Pathogenesis

The pathogenesis of NSAID-induced enteropathy is uncertain, but there have been some recent important advances in its elucidation with the formulation of a two-stage pathogenic framework [70]. First there is specific, if not pathognomic, biochemical damage that leads to ultrastructural alterations, and this is manifested on a tissue level as increased intestinal permeability. The second stage is the consequential nonspecific tissue response which leads to macroscopic damage.

Following ingestion there is a high local concentration of NSAIDs in the small intestine at the site of absorption. NSAIDs cause uncoupling of oxidative phosphorylation of enterocyte mitochondria possibly by virtue of their low pH and high lipid solubility [29, 37, 43, 69, 72]. This leads to two main mechanisms of subcellular damage [70]. First, there is efflux of calcium from mitochondria which leads to a cascade of secondary biochemical events that cause damage via generation of reactive oxygen species. Secondly, the cessation of ATP production leads to loss of regulatory control of intercellular junctions which leads to increased intestinal permeability to luminal substances.

The second stage then follows as the inevitable consequence of increased intestinal permeability. Bile acids further perturbate cell membranes, and a bacterial invasion of the mucosa sets in and this appears to be the main stimulus for neutrophil migration to the intestine [45, 59, 60, 63]. Once the neutrophils find the chemoattractant, the respiratory burst occurs with subsequent internalisation of the chemoattractant and lysosomal enzyme release with indiscriminant damage to the mucosa and hence ulceration, blood and protein loss [32, 49, 68, 79, 80, 82].

Inhibition of prostaglandin production is not a primary event in this framework, as many previous workers have proposed, but is nevertheless important as their inhibition effectively prevents rapid repair of the biochemical damage. Hence the enhanced intestinal permeability is much more prolonged than that seen after alcohol or hypertonicity.

2.2.4 Treatment and Prevention

The dramatic findings of Allison and colleagues [1] that three NSAID users in their series of 713 post-mortem examinations (of which 249 had NSAIDs prescribed during the 6 months before death) had died due to perforation of non specific small intestinal ulcers have recently been published. This emphasises that the problems of NSAID enteropathy can be life threatening. Given the scale of NSAID usage, it is sad to report that there is little concrete information on how to treat established small intestinal enteropathy apart from discontinuing the drugs. This may not be practicable or may lead to a reduction in the quality of the patient's life.

It is clear experimentally that metronidazole or sulphasalazine reduce the small intestinal inflammation [13, 14], but it is not clear whether they obviate the complications to a clinically significant degree. Concomitant prostaglandin administration has been found to protect the gastroduodenal mucosa against NSAID-induced ulceration, but it is not known whether this effect extends to the small intestinal enteropathy. There is an urgent need for studies to address this issue and for a long-term clinical trial to explore whether the drugs shown to offer protection against GI NSAID complications both in the small intestine and in the gastroduodenum exert an overall clinical protective effect in reducing mortality and morbidity.

2.3 Other NSAIDs Small Intestinal Damage

Some of the other reports of NSAID damage of the small intestine may be unrelated to the NSAID enteropathy described above. For example, mefenamic acid and Sulindac have been implicated in a malabsorption syndrome in case reports, with a similar subtotal villous atrophy as found in coeliac disease [27, 35]. Certainly, malabsorption is not normally a feature of NSAID enteropathy, and active and passive transport mechanisms in the small intestinal enterocytes are not affected in the short term by NSAID treatment [12]. It seems likely in these cases that the drugs are producing an idiosyncratic effect on enterocyte differentiation with its attendent consequences on small intestinal morphology and function.

Other effects of NSAIDs are easier to relate to the enteropathy. Indomethacin has been reported to cause intestinal perforation in infants in whom high doses have been used to close a patent ductus arteriosus [2, 52]; here there is an acute effect, which can also be seen in experimental animals. Localised high concentrations of indomethacin in the intestine probably accounted for the complications of Osmosin, an indomethacin preparation which contains potassium bicarbonate as a release agent [22]. The capsules may have adhered to the small intestinal mucosa, and the NSAID damage resulted in perforation. Until recently it was unclear how these effects related to the sort of damage generated by NSAIDs in standard dosage; however, the findings of the post-mortem study described above indicate that perforation is indeed one of the NSAID enteropathy complications, and the effects of Osmosin and high indomethacin concentrations to close patent ductus can be explained on this basis.

3 NSAID Damage of the Gastroduodenal Mucosa

The effects of NSAID damage on the gastroduodenal mucosa are dealt with in detail in another chapter in this volume, but in order to give a balanced view of NSAIDs on the GI tract, we briefly review some of the main points here.

In contrast to the small intestine, where occult inflammation and bleeding occur in over 70 % of patients receiving one of the drugs for 6 months or more, gastroduodenal complications are less common but very dramatic. In long-term studies (>6 months) frank ulceration is seen in about 10 %–30 % of NSAID patients [30, 31, 38, 47]. There is good evidence to show that such ulcers carry a major risk of GI haemorrhage or perforation [33, 34, 38, 63, 71]. Estimates of the risks have been determined, and these depend partly on the design of the study, but a major complication (bleeding or perforation) is expected about once in every 500–800 prescriptions of NSAIDs. This obviously results in a substantial mortality risk (it has been estimated that over 4000 deaths can be attributed to NSAIDs in the United Kingdom annually) and a significant strain on health care resources [6].

In long-term NSAID patients who do not have an ulcer there may nonetheless be endoscopically visible signs of gastroduodenal damage. About 30–50 % of patients have superficial erosions or histological evidence of a type B gastritis.

4 Effects of NSAID on the Colon

Damage to the colon from orally administered NSAIDs is very uncommon, and the literature consists mostly of case reports. NSAIDs may cause an aggressive form of diverticulitis and even perforation; there have been reports of undissolved tablets being found close to perforated diverticulae [16, 19, 20, 26, 73, 75, 84]. In other NSAID patients isolated colonic ulcers have been described [15, 23].

Colonic complications may also ensue from rectal NSAID suppositories [7, 28]. These may be given in the hope of sparing the proximal intestinal mucosa from local NSAID effects, but sadly a significant amount of circulating NSAID is secreted in the bile. Moreover, up to half the patients on NSAID suppositories stop treatment because of pain, irritation, loose motions or rectal bleeding. Such rectal problems may even result in a frank proctitis [48, 81].

There are only a few cases that have been reported of NSAIDs causing a colitis, but it is of interest that these same patients may tolerate other NSAIDs without apparent ill effect [53, 58, 62, 76]. Mefenamates that are in fact weak inhibitors of cyclo-oxygenase are nonetheless frequently associated with diarrhoea, and there are a number of case reports linking their use to a clinically severe colitis which lacks the histopathological severity of classic inflammatory bowel disease in most cases [24–26, 41, 54]. There are some case reports of NSAID-induced relapse of classic inflammatory bowel disease, and these appear to occur within days of receiving the drugs [44, 55, 57].

5 Perspectives

The gastrointestinal effects of NSAIDs are clinically important to doctors practising in a range of specialities and in family practice. We have described in this review that the historical concept of NSAIDs as drugs that specifically damage the gastroduodenal mucosa is incorrect, and that the small intestinal enteropathy causes low-grade inflammation with oozing of blood and protein which may lead to iron deficiency and hypoalbuminaemia, both of which require investigation and treatment. More seriously small intestinal ulceration resulting in perforation, which may be fatal, has also been described. At present it is unclear whether these complications can be effectively prevented by co-prescription of prostaglandins, and as with the gastroduodenal complications a large randomised control trial is clearly needed because of the size of the problem. Further research is also required to understand the cellular and molecular mechanism of the enteropathy. This is important not only because it will lead to new possibilities of therapeutic intervention, but it will also provide insight into the pathogenesis and pathophysiology of other intestinal inflammatory conditions.

References

1. Allison, MC, Howatson, AG, Torrance, CJ, Lee, FD, Russell, RI (1992) Gastro-intestinal damage associated with the use of nonsteroidal anti-inflammatory drugs. N Engl J Med 327: 749–754
2. Alpan, G, Eyal, F, Vinograd, I, Udassin, R, Amir, G, Mogle, P, Glick, B (1985) Localized intestinal perforation after enteral administration of indomethacin in premature infants. J Pediatr 106: 277–281
3. Armstrong, CP, Blower, AL (1987) Nonsteroidal anti-inflammatory drugs and life threatening complications of peptic ulcer disease. Gut 28: 527–532
4. Bahrt, KM, Korman, LY, Nashel, DJ (1984) Significance of a positive test for occult blood in stools of patients taking anti-inflammatory drugs. Arch Intern Med 144: 2165–2166
5. Bartle, WR, Gupta, AK, Lazor, J (1986) Nonsteroidal anti-inflammatory drugs and gastrointestinal bleeding: a case-control study. Arch Intern Med 146: 2365–2367
6. Beardon, PHG, Brown, SV, McDevitt, DG (1989) Gastrointestinal events in patients prescribed NSAIDs: a controlled study using record linkage in Tayside. Q J Med 71: 497–505
7. Berry, H, Seinson, D, Jones, H, Hamilton, EBD (1978) Indomethacin and naproxen suppositories in the treatment of rheumatoid arthritis. Ann Rheum Dis 37: 370–372
8. Bjarnason, I, Williams, P, So, A, Zanelli, G, Levi, AJ, Gumpel, MJ, Peters, TJ, Ansell, B (1984) Intestinal permeability and inflammation in rheumatoid arthritis; effects of nonsteroidal anti-inflammatory drugs. Lancet II: 1171–1174
9. Bjarnason, I, Zanelli, G, Smith, T, Prouse, P, De Lacey, G, Gumpel, MJ, Levi, AJ (1987) Nonsteroidal anti-inflammatory drug induced inflammation in humans. Gastroenterology 93: 480–489
10. Bjarnason, I, Zanelli, G, Prouse, P, Smethurst, P, Smith, T, Levi, S, Gumpel, MJ, Levi, AJ (1987) Blood and protein loss via small intestinal inflammation induced by nonsteroidal anti-inflammatory drugs. Lancet II: 711–714
11. Bjarnason, I, Price, AB, Zanelli, G, Smethurst, P, Burke, M, Gumpel, MJ, Levi, AJ (1988) Clinico-pathological features of NSAID induced small intestinal strictures. Gastroenterology 94: 1070–1074
12. Bjarnason, I, Smethurst, P, Fenn, GC, Lee, CF, Menzies, IS, Levi, AJ (1989) Misoprostol reduces indomethacin induced changes in human small intestinal permeability. Dig Dis Sci 34: 407–411
13. Bjarnason, I, Hopkinson, N, Zanelli, G, Prouse, P, Gumpel, MJ, Levi, AJ (1990) The treatment of nonsteroidal anti-inflammatory drug induced enteropathy. Gut 31: 777–780
14. Bjarnason, I, Hayllar, J, Smethurst, P, Price, AB, Menzies, IS, Gumpel, MJ (1992) Metronidazole reduces inflammation and blood loss in NSAID enteropathy. Gut 33: 1204–1208

15. Bravo, AC, Lowman, RM (1968) Benign ulcer of sigmoid colon. Radiology 90: 113–115
16. Campbell, K, Steele, RJC (1991) Non-steroidal anti-inflammatory drugs and complicated diverticular disease: a case-control study. Br J Surg 78: 190–191
17. Cartwright, GE, Lee, GR (1972) The anaemia of chronic disorder. Br J Haematol 21: 147–152
18. Collins, AJ, A du Toit, J (1987) Upper gastrointestinal findings and faecal occult blood in patients with rheumatic disease taking non-steroidal anti-inflammatory drugs. Br J Rheumatol 26: 295–298
19. Corder, A (1987) Steroids, nonsteroidal anti-inflammatory drugs and serious complications of diverticular disease. Br J Med 295:1238
20. Coutrot, S, Roland, D, Barbier, J, Marcq, PVD, Alcalay, M, Matuchansky, C (1978) Acute perforation of colonic diverticula associated with short term indomethacin. Lancet II: 1055–1056
21. Croft, DN, Wood, PWH (1967) Gastric mucosal and susceptibility to occult gastrointestinal bleeding caused by aspirin. Br Med J I: 137–141
22. Day, TK (1983) Intestinal perforation associated with slow release indomethacin capsules. Br Med J 287: 1671–1672
23. Debenham, GP (1966) Ulcer of the caecum during oxyphenylbutazone (Tanderil) therapy. Can Med Assoc J 94: 1182–1184
24. Doman, DB, Goldberg, HJ (1986) A case of meclofenamate sodium-induced colitis. Am J Gastroenterol 81: 1220–1221
25. Edwards, AL, Heagerty, AM, Bing, RF (1983) Enteritis and colitis associated with mefenamic acid. Br Med J 287: 1627
26. Finkelstein, JA, Jamieson, CG (1987) An association between anti-inflammatory medication and internal pelvic fistulas. Dis Col Rect 30: 168–170
27. Freeman, HJ (1986) Sulindac-associated small bowel lesion. J Clin Gastroenterol 8: 569–571
28. Gizzi, G, Villani, V, Brandi, G, Paganelli, GM, Di Febo, G (1990) Ano-rectal lesions in patients taking suppositories containing non-steroidal anti-inflammatory drugs. Endoscopy 22: 146–248
29. Glanborg-Jorgensen, T, Weis-Fough, US, Neilsen, HH, Olsen, HP (1976) Salicylate and aspirin-induced uncoupling of oxidative phosphorylation in mitochondria isolated from the mucosal membrane of the stomach. Scand J Clin Invest 36: 649–653
30. Graham, DY, Agrawal, NM, Roth, S (1988) Prevention of non-steroidal anti-inflammatory drug induced gastric ulceration with Misoprostol; multicenter, double blind placebo controlled trial. Lancet II: 1277–1280
31. Graham, DY (1990) The relationship between NSAID use and peptic ulcer disease. Gastroenterol Clin N Am 19: 171–182
32. Granger, DN, Benoit, JN, Suzuki, M, Grisham, MB (1985) Leucocyte adherence to venular endothelium during ischemia perfusion. Am J Physiol 257: G 683–G 688
33. Griffin, MR, Ray, WA, Schaffner, W (1988) NSAID use and death from peptic ulcer in the elderly. Ann Intern Med 109: 359–364
34. Griffin, MR, Piper, JM, Dougherty, JR, Snowden, M, Ray, WA (1991) Non-steroidal anti-inflammatory drug use and increased risk for peptic ulcer disease in elderly persons. Ann Intern Med 114: 257–263
35. Hall, RI, Petty, AH, Cobden, I, Lendrum, R (1983) Enteritis and colitis associated with mefenamic acid. Br Med J 287: 1182
36. Hansen, TM, Hansen, NE, Birgens, HS, Holund, B, Lorenzen, I (1983) Serum ferritin and the assessment of iron deficiency in rheumatoid arthritis. Scand J Gastroenterol 12: 353–359
37. Hayllar, J, Somasundaram, S, Sarathchandra, P, Levi AJ, Bjarnason, I (1990) Early cellular events in the pathogenesis of NSAID enteropathy in the rat. Gastroenterology 100: A 216

38. Hayllar, J, MacPherson, A, Bjarnason, I (1992) Gastroprotection and nonsteroidal anti-inflammatory drugs Drug Safety 7: 86–105
39. Hershfield, NB (1992) Endoscopic description of diaphragm disease induced by nonsteroidal anti-inflammatory drugs. Gastroint Endosc 38: 267
40. Huber, T, Ruchti, C, Halter, F (1991) Nonsteroidal antiinflammatory drug-induced colonic strictures: a case report. Gastroenterology 100: 1119–1122
41. Isaacs PET, Sladen, GE, Filpie, I (1987) Mefenamic acid enteropathy. J Clin Pathol 40: 121–127
42. Johnson, F (1987) Recurrent small bowel obstruction with piroxicam. Br J Surg 74: 654
43. Kaedekar, DK (1973) Effects of salicylate and related compounds in gastric HCl secretions. Am J Physiol 225: 521–527
44. Kaufman, HJ, Taubin, HL (1987) NSAID activate quiescent inflammatory bowel disease. Ann Intern Med 107: 513–516
45. Kent, TH, Cardeli RM, Stanler, FU (1969) Small intestinal ulcers and intestinal flora in rats given indomethacin. Am J Pathol 54: 237–245
46. Lang, J, Price AB, Levi AJ, Burk, M, Gumpel, JM, Bjarnason, I (1988) Diaphragm disease: the pathology of non-steroidal anti-inflammatory drug induced small intestinal strictures. J Clin Path 41: 516–526
47. Langman, MJS (1989) Epidemiological evidence on the association between peptic ulceration and antiinflammatory drugs. Gastroenterology 96: 640–646
48. Levy, N, Gaspar, E (1975) Rectal bleeding and indomethacin suppositories. Lancet I: 577
49. Malech, MI, Callin, JI (1987) Neutrophils in human disease. N Eng J Med 317: 687–694
50. Morris, AJ, Madhock, R, Sturrock, RD, Capell, HA, MacKenzie, JF (1991) Enteroscopic diagnosis of small bowel ulceration in patients receiving nonsteroidal anti-inflammatory drugs. Lancet 337: 520
51. Morris, AJ, Wasson, LA, MacKenzie, JF (1992) Small bowel enteroscopy in undiagnosed gastrointestinal blood loss. Gut 33: 887–889
52. Nagaraj, HS, Sandhu, AS, Cook, LN, Buchuno, JT, Groff, DB (1981) Gastrointestinal perforation following indomethacin in very low birth weight infants. J Paediatr Surg 16: 1003–1007
53. Pearson, DJ, Stones, NA, Bentley, SJ, Reid, H (1983) Proctocolitis induced by salicylate and associated with asthma and recurrent nasal polyps. Br Med J 287: 1675
54. Phillips, MS, Fehilly, B, Stewart, S, Dronfield, WM (1983) Enteritis and colitis associated with mefenamic acid. Br Med J 287: 1626–1627
55. Rampton, DS, Sladen, GGE (1981) Relapse of ulcerative proctocolitis during treatment with NSAID. Postgrad Med J 57: 297–299
56. Rampton, DS, Trapping, PJ (1983) Enteritis and colitis associated with mefenamic acid. Br Med J 287: 1627
57. Rampton, DS, McNeil, NI, Sarner, M (1983) Analgesic ingestion and other factors preceding relapse in ulcerative colitis. Gut 24: 187–189
58. Ravi, S, Keat, AC, Keat, ECB (1986) Colitis caused by NSAID. Postgrad Med J 62: 773–776
59. Robert, A (1975) Cytoprotection by prostaglandins. Gastroenterlogy 77: 761–767
60. Robert, A, Asano, T (1977) Resistance of germ free rats to indomethacin-induced intestinal lesions. Prostaglandins 14: 331–341
61. Rooney, PJ, Jenkins, RT, Smith, KM, Coates, G (1986) 111-Indium-labelled polymorphonuclear leucocyte scans in rheumatoid arthritis – an important clinical cause of positive results. Br J Rheumatol 25: 167–170
62. Rutherford, D, Stockdill, G, Hammer-Hodges, DW, Ferguson, A (1984) Proctocolitis induced by salicylates. Br Med J 288: 794
63. Satoh, H, Guth, PH, Grossmann, MI (1983) Role of bacteria in gastric ulceration produced by indomethacin in the rat: cytoprotective action of antibiotics. Gastroenterology 84: 483–489

64. Saverymuttu, SH, Peters, AM, Lavender, JP, Hodgson, HJ, Chadwick, VS (1983) 111-Indium autologous leucocytes in inflammatory bowel disease. Gut 24: 293–299
65. Saverymuttu, SH, Peters, AM, Lavender, JP, Hodgson, H, Chadwick, VS (1983) Quantitative faecal indium-111 labelled leucocyte excretion assessment of disease activity in Chron's disease. Gastroenterology 85: 1333–1339
66. Saverymuttu, SH, Camilleri, M, Rees, H, Cavender, TP, Hodgson, HJF (1986) Indium-111 granulocyte scanning comparison with colonoscopy, histology and faecal indium-111 excretion in assessing disease extent and activity in colitis. Gastroenterology 90: 1121–1128
67. Segal, AW, Isenberg, DA, Hajirousow, V, Tolfree, S, Clark, J, Smaith, ML (1986) Preliminary evidence for gut involvement in the pathogenesis of rheumatoid arthritis? Br J Rheumatol 25: 162–166
68. Segall, AW (1990) The electron transport chain of the microbicidal oxidase of phagocytic cells and its involvement in the molecular pathology of chronic granulomatous disease. In: Peters, TJ (ed) The cell biology of inflammation in the gastrointestinal tract. Corners Publication, Hull, pp 51–73
69. Somasundaram, S, Macpherson, AJ, Hayllar, J, Saratchandra, P, Bjarnason, I (1992) Enterocyte mitochondrial damage due to NSAID in the rat. Gut 33 (Suppl.): S 5
70. Somasundaram, S, Hayllar, J, Macpherson, A, Bjarnason, I (1993) The biochemical basis of NSAID-induced gastrointestinal damage: a review and a hypothesis. To be published
71. Sommerville, K, Faulkner, G, Langman, M (1986) Non-steroidal anti-inflammatory drugs and bleeding peptic ulcer. Lancet I: 462–464
72. Spenny, JG, Bhown, M (1977) Effects of acetylsalicylic acid on gastric mucosa. II. Mucosal ATP and phosphocreatine content and salicylic effects on mitochondrial metabolism. Gastroenterlogy 73: 995–999
73. Stewart, JT, Pennington, CR, Pringle, R (1985) Anti-inflammatory drugs and bowel perforation und haemorrhage. Br Med J 290: 787–788
74. Sukumar, L (1987) Recurrent small bowel obstruction with piroxicam. Br J Surg 74: 186
75. Tancer, ML, Zahiruddin, S (1966) Diagnosis of sigmoidovaginal fistula by vaginogram. Obst Gynecol 28: 815–819
76. Tanner, AR, Raghunat, H (1988) Colonic inflammation and NSAID administration. Digestion 41: 116–120
77. Teahon, K, Webster, D, Price, AB, Levi, AJ, Bjarnason, I (1991) Hypogammaglobulinaemic enteropathy. Gastroenterology 100: A 620
78. Vreudgenhil, G, Wognum, AW, Van Hijk, HG, Swaak, AJG (1990) Anaemia in rheumatoid arthritis: the role of iron, vitamin B 12, for folic acid and eryhtropoietin responsiveness. Ann Rheum Dis 49: 93–98
79. Wallace, JL, Keenan, CM, Granger, DN (1990) Gastric ulceration induced by nonsteroidal anti-inflammatory drugs is a neutrophil dependent process. Am J Physiol 259: G 462–G 467
80. Wallace, JL, Arfors, KE, McKnight, GW (1991) A monoclonal antibody against the CD 18 leucocyte adhesion molecule prevents indomethacin-induced gastric damage in the rabbit. Gastroenterology 100: 878–883
81. Walls, J, Bell, D, Schora, W (1968) Rectal bleeding and indomethacin. Br Med J I: 52
82. Weiss, SJ (1989) Tissue destruction by neutrophils N. Engl J Med 320: 365–376
83. Wilkinson, PC (1990) Leucocyte locomotion: determinants of locomotor capacity, chemotaxis and chemokinesis. In: Peters, TJ (ed) The cell biology of inflammation in the gastrointestinal tract. Corners Publication, Hull, pp 15–27
84. Wilson, RG, Smith, AN, MacIntyre, IMC (1990) Complications of diverticular disease and nonsteroidal anti-inflammatory drugs: a prospective study. Br J Surg 77: 1103–1104

Drug-Induced Malabsorption

T. WEHRMANN, B. LEMBCKE, AND W. F. CASPARY

Abteilung für Gastroenterologie, Fakultät für Klinische Medizin,
Universität Heidelberg, Mannheim, BRD

1 Introduction

1.1 General Aspects

Drugs may induce malassimilation of nutrients by direct or indirect, specific or non specific modes of action. It is important to distinguish first between the interference of drugs with the process of digestion or absorption since an increased loss of nutrients in the stool may be caused by a derangement of either or both functions. These side effects may be induced by a variety of chemically totally different compounds and may be independent of the route of drug administration (enteral or parentereral), while excretion of drugs (or their metabolites) in gut secretions and bile accounts for the interference with nutrient absorption even after parenteral administration. However, the clinical relevance of the different pathophysiological mechanisms merits careful interpretation. Apart from the clinical importance of adverse drug reactions, the therapeutic potential of inhibiting digestive and absorptive gastrointestinal functions in the treatment of diabetes mellitus (acarbose), hyperlipidaemia (cholestyramine), and dumping syndrome (guar, so called "gelling agents") had been established. For the purpose of this review, the effects of drugs on the gastrointestinal absorptive function are structured according to six different underlying pathophysiological mechanisms [88] (Table 1).

Table 1. Pathophysiology of adverse drug reactions causing malabsorption

Direct mucosal toxicity	Colchicine, cytostatics, antibiotics (neomycin)
Inhibition of hydrolytic enzymes	Guar, pectins, acarbose, α-amylase inhibitors, salazosulfapyridine, phenytoin
Inhibition of active transport	Biguanides fenfluramine, prenylamine
Physicochemical interference	Cholestyramine, neomycin, antacids
Inhibition of "preintestinal" digestive process	Ocreotide, tendamistate
Modification of gastrointestinal motility	Metoclopramide, cisapride, domperidone, erythromycin

1.2 Symptoms of Drug-Induced Malabsorption

Commonly, symptoms of drug-induced malabsorption reach clinical relevance only after prolonged use of the pharmacological agent in question. The malabsorption of substrates may be clinically inapparent over a long period, either because of a storage capacity of the substrate (e. g., vitamin B_{12}) or incomplete inhibition of the digestive or absorptive process. When this functional reserve capacity is depleted, symptoms of malabsorption develop depending on the nutritional deficiency. The malabsorption process by itself (e.g., vitamin B_{12} or folic acid) may remain asymptomatic. On the other hand, compounds causing immediate cellular injury (e.g., methotrexate) or inhibition of brush-border enzymes result in unequivocal symptoms of either carbohydrate (diarrhea, flatulence, burbulence) or fat (steathorrhea, weight loss) malabsorption as a rapid response following drug administration. The clinical presentation of drug-induced malabsorption may thus be obvious mimic other conditions. Therefore, we believe it most helpful to present the data available on this field in the context of the underlying pathophysiological processes (Table 1).

2 Direct Mucosal Toxicity

2.1 Pathophysiology

Drugs with direct toxic effects on the mucosa which lead to alterations of the normal mucosal architecture may induce the so-called "secondary" malabsorption. Formerly, treatment of hyperlipidemia with tripiranol caused intestinal mucosal damage which induced carbohydrate and fat malabsorption [109]. Today, secondary malabsorption due to treatment of malign diseases with cytostatic agents is a well-known phenomenon. Diarrhea is particularly common during treatment with antimetabolites such as methotrexate, 5-fluorouracil, and cytosine arabinoside or antineoplasmatic antibiotics such as actinomycin D and doxorubicin [37]. These cytostatic drugs induce disruption of intestinal mucosal cell membranes or intracellularly of nuclear DNA and may have direct effects on intracellular enzymes by denaturation or competitive inhibition [4]. Moreover, small-intestinal transport processes and mucosal enzyme synthesis may be affected by these agents [70]. For patients on treatment with drugs known to have such direct or indirect mucosal toxicity, periodic evaluations of mucosal function or morphology are therefore suggested if symptoms of malabsorption occur.

2.2 Colchicine

As with the vinca alkaloids, colchicine administration causes impaired cell division by metaphasic arrest occurring 1–6 h after ingestion of the compound [68]. Therefore diarrhea and malabsorption of nutrients are frequent but reversible consequences of short-term administration of large doses of colchicine. However, experimental evidence in animals and humans indicates that doses of colchicine too small to affect the mitotic rate of crypt cells may impair mucosal enzyme synthesis [33, 73, 110]. In humans, ingestion of 1.9–3.9 mg colchicine daily has been shown to cause minimal histological changes which correlate poorly with significantly decreased jejunal disaccharidase activities and laboratory parameters of carbohydrate and fat malabsorption [57, 106, 115]. The effect of colchicine on carbohydrate absorption has been demonstrated to be dose dependent since 38 % of patients taking 1.9 mg daily and 72 % of those taking 3.9 mg showed carbohydrate malabsorption by the D-xylose test [106]. Long-term administration of small doses of colchicine for treatment of recurrent polyserositis ("Mediterranean fever") induced only mild steatorrhea and a minor decrease in the jejunal Na^+K^+-ATPase activity [46]. In a few reported cases where fatal outcome occurred after long-term colchicine administration for prophylaxis of gout exacerbation, diffuse mucosal damage attributable to drug toxicity was demonstrated [124].

2.3 Cytostatics

2.3.1 Methotrexate

This compound inhibits dihydrofolate reductase activity and thus prevents DNA replication by depleting the active coenzyme tetrahydrofolic acid. In addition to the powerfully inhibiting action on folate reductase, methotrexate has also been shown to interfere with intestinal folate transport [31]. In the rat, methotrexate depressed metabolic activity of the gut mucosa [111]. Therefore, mucosal damage was inevitably observed in humans since the small intestinal mucosa is a rapidly proliferating tissue [45]. It was suggested that methotrexate induced mucosal damage by direct and indirect effects on the enterocyte [103]. Apart from the prevention of folic acid absorption by competitive enzyme inhibition (see above), the carbohydrate, fat, vitamin B_{12}, and vitamin K malabsorption after methotrexate is considered to result from structural alterations of the intestinal mucosa [36, 129]. Capel et al. [16] demonstrated an increase in passive permeation of the mucosal membrane barrier after methotrexate administration in the rat, whereas Robinson et al. [111] showed an inhibition of active jejunal sugar and amino acid transport processes.

2.3.2 5-Fluorouracil

It has been demonstrated that 5-fluorouracil has the same potential as methotrexate to induce strong mucosal damage and secondary malabsorption [93]. Therefore, a close correlation between the decrease in intestinal glucose absorption and the loss of intestinal villous cells has been found after single administration of 5-fluorouracil [112].

2.3.3 Mitomycin C

Recently Mizuno [99] showed that mitomycin C, like other alkylating agents, inhibits active glucose transport systems of the intestinal mucosa. However, passive permeability of glucose increased simultaneously. Therefore it was speculated that the adverse effect of the drug on glucose uptake was secondary to the antimitotic activity of the compound and not related to the inhibition of the membrane glucose carrier system since this inhibition was demonstrable only after long-term treatment and not during short-term incubations in vitro.

2.3.4 Doxorubicin and Actinomycin

Cytostatics with protein synthesis inhibitor action such as the antibiotics doxorubicin and actinomycin, have been shown to impair the intestinal mucosal transport of amino acids and sugars and to reduce the activity of brush-border enzymes such as hydrolases and disaccharidases [60, 71]. The most likely mechanism to induce these adverse effects is a decrease in brush-border carrier proteins and enzymes, but direct mucosal damage may also occur. These effects should be considered especially in patients receiving high-calory, milk-containing solutions for nutritional support under chemotherapy [88].

2.4 Antibiotics

Compounds with inhibitory action on bacterial protein synthesis (e.g., neomycin, kanamycin, paromycin, tetracycline) and substances which interfere with the structural integrity of bacterial membranes (e.g., polymyxin, bacitracin) reveal malabsorptive side effects that are partially related to mucosal damage [53, 56, 80, 117, 123].

2.4.1 Neomycin

Neomycin is a polybasic aminoglycoside used for the treatment of hyperammonemia states to prevent hepatic encephalopathy and spontaneous bacterial peritonitis. It is known to induce the clinically most important malabsorption syndrome among antibiotics. Despite the fact that neomycin is poorly absorbed from the gastrointestinal tract after oral administration, the compound induces a dose-dependent, reversible malabsorption of fat, cholesterol, carotene, D-xylose, glucose, some vitamins, and electrolytes [1, 3, 43, 56, 78, 118]. The drug-induced malabsorption of fat may cause vitamin K malabsorption, particularly after prolonged administration [54]. The pathophysiological mechanism responsible for this mode of action seems to be complex; using higher doses of neomycin (6–12 g per day) serious mucosal damage of the intestine has been confirmed histologically [43, 80]. However, significant fat malabsorption was also described without histological mucosal injury [101]. For the cholesterol-lowering effect of neomycin, the ability of the compound to precipitate bile acids and micellar fatty acids and the potency of neomycin to induce crypt cell injury, which may lead to a reduced cholesterol synthesis in the crypt cell region, were suggested as underlying pathophysiological mechanisms [40, 55, 127]. The observed carbohydrate malabsorption during long-term neomycin administration can be attributed both to the reduction of monosaccharide absorption [80, 101] and to the inhibition of small intestinal lactase activity [101]. Lembcke and Caspary [87] showed an unequivocally flattened lactose tolerance curve and a rise in breath hydrogen concentration after neomycin administration to healthy volunteers. A significant malabsorption of sucrose was not observed. These findings indicate that neomycin does not inhibit bacterial metabolism of (malabsorbed) carbohydrates in the human colon by which both hydrogen and short-chain fatty acids are produced [88]. Since fecal acidification due to malabsorption of carbohydrates may lead to a beneficial shift in colonic ammonia metabolism [131], this mode of action of neomycin may be regarded not as a side effect of the drug, but as an additional therapeutic effect of the compound in hyperammonia states. However, parenteral intramuscular administration of neomycin, presumably comparable to the portion of the drug absorbed (3 %), did not cause carbohydrate or fat malabsorption [92].

3 Inhibition of Hydrolytic Enzymes

3.1 Pathophysiology

Carbohydrates normally represent the majority of caloric ingestion of human diet. As mono-, oligo-, and especially polysaccharides they form not only the largest proportion quantitatively but also the main energy supply in humans. Oligo- and polysaccharides are not absorbed to any appreciable amount in the small intestine. To be absorbed they must first be broken down to monosaccharides. Therefore, the first step is cleavage of starch by α-amylase; the second step is cleavage of short-chain oligo- or polysaccharides by membrane-bound hydrolytic enzymes of the small-intestinal mucosa (maltase, sucrase, glucoamylase, trehalase, lactase). The end products of this enzymatic hydrolysis are primarily the monosaccharides glucose, galactose, and fructose. Interference of drugs with this process of enzymatic brush-border membrane hydrolysis leads to malabsorption of carbohydrates.

3.2 Carbohydrate Gelling Agents

It has been found that various non digestible plant polysaccharides (so-called carbohydrate gelling agents or "dietary fiber") such as guar or pectin, due to their physicochemical properties, exert an inhibitory effect on the digestive and absorptive processes in the small intestine [51]. These compounds do not affect the hydrolysis of disaccharidases or dipeptides in homogenates of small-intestinal mucosa in vitro, but when hydrolysis is studied in segments of rat jejunum, the inhibitory effect on membrane hydrolysis is observed. This inhibitory effect seems to be a clue to an increase of the "unstirred water layer," a luminal diffusion barrier covering the surface of the small intestinal mucosa [50]. This mechanism may partially contribute to the desirable effects of this type of fiber supplement, but it appears insufficient to induce malabsorption of nutrients even during long-term administration.

However, it seems to be more important that the viscosity-related increase in the luminal barrier may lead to a retardation of intestinal uptake of nutrients. In vitro and in vivo studies have shown that the therapeutic effect of delaying absorption may be related to their effect on the "unstirred layer resistance" [8, 36, 49, 52, 58]. However, both carbohydrate gelling agents (e. g., guar) and phytate-containing fiber preparations (e. g., bran) may diminish the absorption of minerals and iron [69, 83, 107].

Nutrient malabsorption can be compensated by a shift to the more distal absorption sites and adaptive growth of the distal gut; however, no such mechanisms exist for compensation of reduced bile acid absorption in the ileum. This renders bile acid malabsorption a possibly important mechanism for the cholesterol-lowering effects of guar [47, 82]. The long-term clinical importance of these effects is not known.

3.3 α-Glucosidase Inhibitors

Besides drug-induced malabsorption as a side effect, the therapeutic rationale of inhibiting carbohydrate absorptive function of the gastrointestinal tract has been finally established by development of α-Glucosidase inhibitors [32]. The most potent and practical way to reduce or modulate carbohydrate absorption is by acarbose, which has a 15,000-fold higher affinity for sucrase than for the natural substrate of the enzyme, sucrose [21, 27]. Acarbose exerts its effect through competitive inhibition of human α-glucosidases with a rank order of inhibitory potency on glucoamylase > sucrase > maltase > isomaltase. The compound has little or no effect on trehalase and lactase activity [21]. The drug has been proven to offer a promising auxiliary treatment alternative in patients with insulin-dependent or non-insulin-dependent diabetes mellitus [20, 38, 41]. Further, the compound has been investigated for the treatment of hyperlipoproteinemia and the dumping syndrome [38]. Perfusion experiments in humans have shown that acarbose not only inhibits the absorption of carbohydrates but also inhibits net sodium and water absorption from the small intestine [27]. This inhibitor does not alter the absorption of monosaccharides, but pancreatic α-amylase is inhibited to some extent [105].

Carbohydrate malabsorption, even at minimal levels can be detected by recording breath hydrogen (H_2) exhalation after a carbohydrate load [87]. This parameter theoretically enables an effective dosage level to be established at which clinical important malabsorption does not occur [88].

For clinical purposes it is noteworthy that symptoms of carbohydrate malabsorption (bloating, flatulence, diarrhea) may subside during long-term administration of acarbose, although the therapeutic effect (flattening of the postprandial blood glucose level and the hormone response) remains unchanged [59]. It has been reported that only 5 % of patients discontinued acarbose treatment during long-term administration [2]. However, low-dose regimens appear to be the most fruitful approach to the effective reduction of postprandial hyperglycemia without unpleasant symptoms of carbohydrate malabsorption [86].

Besides acarbose, other inhibitors of α-glucosidase activity have been tested: BAY O 1099 (Miglitol, Bayer, Germany), BAY M 1248 (Emiglate, Bayer, Germany), and other, nitrogen-containing monosaccharides (e. g., AO-128, Takeda, Japan, and MDL 25637, Merrell Dow, USA). However, carbohydrate malabsorption still remains the basic feature of their common mode of action, and cannot be regarded as specific to any of these compounds [90].

3.4 α-Amylase Inhibitors

Pancreatic secretory insufficiency due to chronic pancreatis or resection of the pancreas leads to maldigestion and thus malabsorption of nutrients. Several attemps have been made to modulate the rate of intestinal carbohydrate absorption by using inhibitors of α-amylase activity. Therefore, this naturally occurring principle has been rediscovered for use to reduce the glycemic response to starch ingestion [105]. Several α-amylase inhibitors (tendamistate, trestatin, phaseolamin and derivates) have been investigated in patients [48, 84, 98], but none has yet been approved for therapeutic use. Like acarbose, these compounds may flatten the postprandial blood glucose level and induce moderate symptoms of carbohydrate malabsorption [12]. There have been attempts in the United States to misuse α-amylase inhibitors ("starch blocker") to achieve weight reduction; however, these have been unsuccessful [13] since efficient reabsorption of short-chain fatty acids in the colon salvages calories in carbohydrate malabsorption states [14].

3.5 Sulfasalazine

After oral ingestion of folate, in the form of pteroylpolyglutamates, this substrate is hydrolyzed by a specific brush-border peptidase (folate conjugase or pteroylpolyglutamase) to pteroylmonoglutamate. This process is highly pH-sensitive and does not depend on the subsequent metabolic steps of mucosal reduction (dihydrofolate reductase) and methylation.

Methyltetrahydrofolate is the principal intestinal product among several folate derivatives. It has been demonstrated by Reisenauer and Halsted [108] that sulfasalazine, using partially purified brush-border pteroylpolyglutamate hydrolase (folate conjugase), is a competitive inhibitor of this enzymatic hydrolization. No similar inhibitory potency has been found for 5-aminosalicyclic acid, sulfapyridine, ethanol, or phenytoin. Moreover, sulfasalazine inhibits folate absorption, irrespective of whether the substrate is the mono- or polyglutamate, or whether it is in the reduced state [113]. Kinetic experiments on folate transport in vitro displayed a competitive inhibition of the folate transport carrier by sulfasalazine [133]. These findings have clinical importance in the long-term treatment of Crohn's disease and ulcerative colitis by inducing megaloblastic anemia due to folate deficiency.

3.6 Phenytoin

The pathophysiology of folate malabsorption during anticonvulsant therapy with phenytoin is not yet fully understood. Formerly, competitive inhibition of folate conjugase was suggested by several authors [5, 77, 114], while recent data from Reisenauer and Halsted [108] provide a strong argument against any effect of phenytoin on this enzyme. Further, no effect of phenytoin on folate transport in vitro or on folate deficiency attributable to a pH reduction by the compound was detected by Zimmerman et al. [133]. The most likely mechanism by which phenytoin may induce folate depletion is by unspecific induction of hepatic enzymes, thereby accelerating folate metabolism [97]. Analogous to the effect on folate metabolism, phenytoin has been shown to inhibit small-intestinal calcium absorption [18]. Further, it was demonstrated that this effect on calcium uptake was reversible 20 days after drug withdrawal [18]. This selective inhibitory action is currently interpreted as being due to induction of the activity of the hepatic drug-metabolizing enzyme system (like its effect on folate metabolism) and accelerated vitamin D metabolism after phenytoin treatment, resulting in exaggerated hydroxylation of vitamin D_3 to 25-hydroxycholecalciferol (25-HOCC), followed by biliary secretion. Thus a depletion of both 25-HOCC and the active form of vitamin D (1,25-dihydroxycholecalciferol) ensues [28, 66]. Thus, the frequent finding of impaired calcium absorption under long-term phenytoin administration can be corrected by vitamin D substitution [28].

4 Inhibition of Active Transport

4.1 Pathophysiology

Due to the large reserve capacity of the small bowel and the adaptional properties of the distal gut, only strong and relevant pharmacological inhibition of active transport results in adverse effects. Among the drugs currently used for pharmacotherapy few have any clinical relevant effect on intestinal transport.

4.2 Biguanides

Biguanides have been shown to be effective in the treatment of non-insulin-dependent diabetes mellitus and the dumping syndrome [7, 29, 65]. In addition to metabolic effects upon glucose utilization in muscle tissue, inhibition of gluconeogenesis, retardation of gastric emptying, and anorectic properties, biguanides have been recognized in experimental studies to interfere with active intestinal glucose transport [7, 9, 29, 65]. However, using breath hydrogen analysis, Olsen [100] was not able to detect any significant malabsorption or carbohydrates after phenformin administration in humans. Thus, the observed influence of phenformin on intestinal active transport processes in vitro probably results in delayed rather than incomplete glucose absorption [88]. In addition to this effect of biguanides on glucose uptake, it has been demonstrated that small-intestinal absorption of various amino acids [24], calcium [17], bile acids [25], and dipeptides [85] is reduced after biguanide administration in experimental studies. Further, both phenformin and metformin may evoke malabsorption of vitamin B_{12} at therapeutic dosages in humans [6, 39, 128]. In diabetic patients, however, neither these two biguanides nor buformin induces bile acid malabsorption or steatorrhea, but bacterial overgrowth is observed after metformin administration [19]. This mechanism may also be regarded as responsible for vitamin B_{12} malabsorption during biguanide therapy [6, 39, 128].

4.3 Fenfluramine

Fenfluramine is an anorexigenic drug which primarily affects satiety by central nervous mechanisms [10]. Loose stools are a frequent adverse effect of this compound [76], but the underlying mechanisms have not yet been fully elucidated. Lembcke and Caspary [88] have shown that fenfluramine is an inhibitor (from the luminal side) of active sugar, amino acid, and bile acid transport in the small intestine. However, in humans after an oral carbohydrate load, reduced blood glucose increments in response to fenfluramine administration are not associated with an increase in breath hydrogen exhalation over 3 h [88]. Fenfluramine, as the biguanides, appears to retard glucose absorption, but this mechanism does not seem to contribute to the gastrointestinal side effects of this compound.

4.4 Prenylamine

The calcium antagonist prenylamine has been reported to be useful in controlling symptoms of the dumping syndrome [125] but has not become standard therapy. Since the compound inhibits the active transport of sugars and amino acids in the intestine [23], this may explain the beneficial effect on glucose absorption in patients with dumping syndrome. Using intestinal perfusion techniques, the inhibitory effect of this drug on glucose absorption has also been demonstrated in humans [62].

5 Physicochemical Interference

5.1 Pathophysiology

The adverse effects of some drugs on small-intestinal absorption can be characterized as intraluminal, physicochemical events such as solubilization, chelation, formation of insoluble products, adsorption, and complexation. Such mechanisms have been extensively studied from the viewpoint of drug – drug interactions (e. g., tetracyclines and iron), but the principle also applies to drug-induced malabsorption syndromes. Special binding properties of the drug to some nutrients and precipitation of bile and fatty acids by the compound may be the most important mechanisms causing these side effects.

5.2 Cholestyramine

Cholestyramine interrupts the enterohepatic circulation of bile acids by special anion exchange that binds bile acids within the intestinal lumen.

The drug is used in the treatment of hyperlipoproteinemia, bile acid-induced diarrhea, pruritus due to biliary obstruction or liver disease, and formerly for the treatment of digitoxin overdosage.

As a consequence of bile acid sequestration by cholestyramine, the compound leads to constipation as well as fat malabsorption, which is only slight in patients with intact enterohepatic bile acid pool. Cholestyramine treatment of patients with preexisting bile acid malabsorption (as in cholerrheic enteropathy), however, results inevitably in a significant increase in steatorrhea. Subsequently, malabsorption and depletion of fat soluble vitamins (A, D, E, and K) can occur, and severe complications such as hemorrhage due to hypoprothrombinemia [63] or osteomalacia [72] may result. Cholestyramine may also bind and inhibit the absorption of folic acid [132], vitamin B_{12}, and iron [126].

5.3 Antacids

Most of the frequently used antacid preparations contain aluminum and/or magnesium hydroxide, which inhibits absorption of dietary phosphate by physicochemical binding. Therefore, hypophosphatemia may occur shortly after commencement of antacid therapy, especially if the patient is on a low-phosphate diet [120]. Prolonged antacid administration may therefore result in a phosphate depletion syndrome characterized by hypophosphatemia, hypophosphaturia, hypercalciuria, nephrolithiasis, osteomalacia, muscle weakness, and anorexia [34, 79, 94, 121]. Lembcke et al. [91] however, observed no significant decrease of the serum phosphate level or increase in urinary calcium excretion after a 4-week antacid administration (containing 2.5 g aluminum and 3.5 g magnesium daily) in healthy volunteers.

Antacids may also reduce the absorption of iron, as Hall [67] has shown in patients receiving magnesium trisilicate. Further, a significant decrease in the bioavailability of tetracyclines (tetracycline, oxytetracycline, doxycycline) and chinolones (norfloxacin, ofloxacin, ciprofloxacin) was observed after simultaneous administration with antacids [61, 74]. The data concerning interactions of antacids with the intestinal absorption of β-blockers and digoxin showed discrepant results, thus indicating that significant interaction between antacids and these substances must not be considered as clinically important. However, Mantylä et al. [96] have shown that simultaneous ingestion of antacids and captopril significantly decrease the bioavailability of captopril. Several studies [11, 64, 122] have demonstrated an influence of high-dose antacid preparations on the absorption of H_2 antagonists, whereas (the more frequently used) low-dose antacid preparations fail to decrease the bioavailability of cimetidine [119]. In clinically used dosages of antacid preparations, the well-documented property of antacids to adsorb bile acids in the gastric mucosa [26, 35] may not lead to a bile acid-induced diarrhea.

5.4 Potassium Preparations

Diminished vitamin B_{12} absorption has been found to be an adverse effect of slow-release KCl preparations; this has been contributed to ileal acidification [102]. It is known that the ileal uptake of vitamin B_{12} is pH dependent because the attachment of the cobalamin intrinsic factor complex to the ileal receptor requires a pH above 5.6 [95].

6 Inhibition of "Preintestinal" Digestive Processes

6.1 Pathophysiology

Carbohydrate malabsorption in response to inhibitors of pancreatic α-amylase activity is mentioned above. Similarly, several inhibitors of pancreatic lipase activity have been investigated, but none is currently under consideration for clinical therapy [105].

6.2 Ocreotide

The long-acting somatostatin analogue ocreotide offers therapeutic progress in treatment of somatostatin-sensitive diseases, such as endocrine gastrointestinal tumors (e.g., carcinoid syndrome) and acromegaly. This agent has complex and manifold actions on the digestive tract which may result in fat malabsorption due to impaired endogenous stimulation both of exocrine pancreatic function and gallbladder contractile activity [86]. Theoretically, additional effects on nutrient absorption may occur due to motility-affecting properties of somatostatin: dose-dependent acceleration of gastric emptying, inhibition (lower doses) or stimulation (higher doses) of interdigestive small intestinal motility.

7 Drug-Induced Malabsorption due to Modification of Gastrointestinal Motility

7.1 Pathophysiology

The motility of the gastrointestinal tract is responsible for nutrients being properly exposed to digestive secretory enzymes, bile acids, and the digestive-absorptive surface of the small bowel. Motility also prevents overflushing of the small intestine and of the colon with nutrients. Therefore, gastrointestinal motility seems to determine the rate of absorption of nutrients to an important extent, whereby the most crucial factor may be the rate of gastric emptying. Small bowel motility also plays an important role for the rate and completeness of nutrient absorption due to allowing enough contact time for terminal membrane digestion and absorption. Small-bowel motility interacts closely with secretory and absorptive processes as well as neurohumoral regulation. Surprisingly, while there are numerous studies concerning the effects of delayed or accelerated gastric emptying and intestinal passage on drug concentration and bioavailability, there is only little evidence of pharmacologically modified intestinal motility as a source of malabsorption.

7.2 Prokinetics

While the traditional antidopaminergic agents, such as metoclopramide and domperidone, exert their effects mainly on the upper gut, it has been substantiated that the more recently developed compound cisapride may also have motility-stimulating properties in the lower parts of the gastrointestinal tract. Holgate and Read [75] found no carbohydrate malabsorption in humans after accelerating small-intestinal transit with metoclopramide. If rapid transit was induced by an increased osmotic load ($MgSO_4$), however, the "intestinal hurry" did facilitate carbohydrate malabsorption. Cholesterol absorption, however, is more likely to be affected, since only 20–60 % of a given dose [15] is absorbed under physiological conditions; acceleration of small-intestinal transit may therefore evoke significant malabsorption of dietary cholesterol [104]. In recent years, the strong prokinetic effect of erythromycin and its 14-member lactone ring analogues on antroduodenal motility has been established by several investigators [81, 116]. Ebert et al. [44] demonstrated that erythromycin, in contrast to cisapride, not only accelerates gastric emptying but also delays the postprandial blood glucose rise after feeding in healthy volunteers. This may be due to an effect of the compound on glucose absorption, independent of the motility stimulation, since the secretion of GIP was significantly decreased after erythromycin. Whether this is clinically relevant in the treatment of diabetic gastroparesis with erythromycin must be determined by future studies.

7.3 Drug-Induced-Inhibition of Gastrointestinal Motility

Chronic motility disorders due to long-standing pharmacological inhibition of small-intestinal peristalsis (e. g., treating psychiatric illness with anticholinergic drugs) favor the proliferation of micro-organisms [42] and may result in the small-bowel bacterial overgrowth syndrome. This may be of particular relevance in elderly patients receiving mono-amino-oxidase inhibitors or tricyclic antidepressants.

Clinical features of the bacterial overgrowth syndrome (weight loss, macrocytic anemia, general malaise) are unspecific, occur slowly, and can thus be misinterpreted or, in the case of steatorrhea, not be diagnosed unless specific investigations are performed, or gross abnormalities ensue. Even constipation does not exclude the bacterial overgrowth syndrome, especially if caused by anticholinergic effects [88].

References

1. Asatoor, AM, Chamberlain, MJ, Emmerson, BT, Johnson, JR, Levi, AJ, Milne, MD (1967) metabolic effects of oral neomycin. Clin Sci 33: 111–124
2. Aubell, R, Boehme, K, Berchtold, P (1983) Blood glucose concentrations and glycosuria during and after one year of acarbose therapy. Arzneimittel Forschung 33: 1314–1318
3. Barrowman, JA, D'Mello, A, Herxheimer, A (1973) A single dose of neomycin impairs absorption of vitamin A (retinol) in man. Europ J Clin Pharmacol 5: 199–201
4. Bartelink, A (1972) Drug induced diseases of the gastrointestinal tract. In: Meyler, L, Peck, HM (eds) Drug-induced diseases, vol. 4. Excerpta Medica, Amsterdam, pp 403–422
5. Baugh, CM, Krumdieck, CL (1969) Effect of phenytoin on folic acid conjugases in man. Lancet ii: 512–521
6. Berchtold, P, Bolli, P, Arbenz, H (1969) Intestinale Absorptionsstörung infolge Metforminbehandlung. Diabetologia 5: 405 (Abstract)
7. Biro, L, Banyasz, T, Kovacs, MB, Bajor, M (1961) Die Wirkung des Phenyläthylbiguanids auf die Glukoseresorption. Klin Wochenschr 39: 760–762
8. Blackburn, NA, Redfern, JS, Jarjis, H (1984) The mechanism of action of guar gum in improving glucose tolerance in man. Clin Sci 66: 329–336
9. Bloch, R, Menge, H, Schaarschmidt, WD, Müller, M, Creutzfeldt, W (1973) Biochemische, histochemische, histologische und funktionelle Untersuchungen zur Phenforminwirkung auf die Dünndarmschleimhaut bei Ratte und Mensch. Klin Wochenschr 51: 235–241
10. Blundell, JE, Catham, CJ, Moniz, E, Mcarthur, RA, Rogers, PJ (1979) Structural analysis of the actions of amphetamine and fenfluramine on food intake and feeding behaviour in animals and in man. Curr Med Res Opinion 6 (suppl. 1): 34–54
11. Bodemar, G, Norlander, B, Walen, A (1979) Diminished absorption of cimetidine caused by antacids. Lancet i: 444–445
12. Boivin, M, Flourie, B, Rizz, GA, Go, VLW, DiMagno, EP (1988) Gastrointestinal and metabolic effects of amylase inhibition in diabetics. Gastroenterology 94: 387–391
13. Bo-Linn, GW, Santa Ana, CA, Morawski, SG, Fordtran, JS (1982) Starch Blockers – their effect on calorie absorption from a high-starch meal. N Engl J Med 307: 1413–1416
14. Bond, JH, Levitt, MD (1976) Fate of soluble carbohydrate in the colon of rats and man. J Clin Invest 57: 1158–1164
15. Borgström, B (1969) Quantification of cholesterol absorption in man by fecal analysis after the feeding of a single-isotope labelled meal. J Lipid Res 10: 331–337
16. Capel, ID, Pinnock, MH, Williams, DC (1979) Methotrexate increase passive permeation of the mucosal membrane barrier in the rat. Eur J Clin Oncology Cancer 15: 127–131

17. Caspary, WF (1971) Effect of biguanides on intestinal transport of sugars, amino acids and calcium. Naunyn Schmiederbergs Arch Pharmacol 269: 421–422
18. Caspary, WF (1972) Inhibition of calcium transport by diphenylhydantoin in rat duodenum. Naunyn Schmiedebergs Arch Pharmacol 274: 146–153
19. Caspary, WF (1977) Biguanides and intestinal absorption. Acta Hepato Gastroenterol 24: 473–480
20. Caspary, WF (1985) Diabetes mellitus: Verzögerung der Kohlenhydrat-Resorption als therapeutisches Prinzip. Dtsch Ärztebl 82: 1424–1428
21. Caspary, WF (1990) Interruption of the entero-pancreatic axis: effects of induced malabsorption. Europ J Clin Invest 20 (suppl. 1): 58–64
22. Caspary, WF, Creutzfeldt, W (1971) Analysis of the inhibitory effect of biguanides on glucose absorption. Inhibition of active sugar transport. Diabetologia 7: 379 (abstract)
23. Caspary, WF, Creutzfeldt, W (1972) Hemmung der intestinalen von Zuckern und Aminosäuren durch Prenylamin (Segontin). Dtsch Med Wochenschr 97: 394–396
24. Caspary, WF, Creutzfeldt, W (1973) Inhibition of intestinal amino acid transport by blood sugar lowering biguanides. Diabetologia 9: 6–12
25. Caspary, WF, Creutzfeldt, W (1975) Inhibition of bile salt absorption by blood sugar lowering biguanides. Diabetologia 11: 113–117
26. Caspary, WF, Graf, S (1978) Bindung von Gallensäuren an Antacida. Dtsch Med Wochenschr 103: 825–827
27. Caspary, WF, Kalisch, H (1979) Effect of α-glucosedehydrolase inhibition on intestinal absorption of sucrose, water and sodium in man. Gut 20: 750–755
28. Caspary, WF, Hesch, RD, Matte, R, Ritter, H, Kattermann, R, Emrich, D (1974) Therapie der Calciumresorptionsstörung unter antiepileptischer Behandlung mit 25-hydroxycholecalciferol (25-OH-CC). Verh Dtsch Ges Inn Med 80: 1277–1280
29. Caspary, WF, Zavada, I, Reimold, V, Graf, S, Creutzfeldt, W (1977) Alteration of bile acid metabolism and vitamin B_{12} absorption in diabetics on biguanides. Diabetologia 13: 187–193
30. Caspary, WF, Elsenhans, B, Süfke, U, Graf, S, Creutzfeldt, W (1980) Effect of dietary fiber on absorption and motility. Front Hormone Res 7: 202–207
31. Chungi, VS, Bourne, DW, Dittert, LW (1979) Competitive inhibition between folic acid and methotrexate for transport carrier in the rat small intestine. J Pharmaceut Sci 68: 1552–1553
32. Clissold, SP, Edwards, C (1991) Acarbose. A preliminary review of its pharmacodynamic and pharmacokinetic properties, and therapeutic potential. Drugs 35: 214–243
33. Cohen, MI, McNamara, H (1970) The effect of colchicine on guinea pig intestinal enzyme activity. Am J Dig Dis 15: 247–250
34. Cooke, N, Teitelbaum, S, Avioli, LV (1978) Antacid-induced osteomalacia and nephrolithiasis. Arch Intern Med 138: 1007–1009
35. Cousar, CD, Gadacz, TR (1981) Comparison of antacids on the binding of bile salts. Gastroenterology 80: 1357–1360
36. Craft, AW, Kay, HEM, Lawson, DN, McElwein, TJ (1977) Methotrexate-induced malabsorption in children with acute lymphoblastic leucaemia. Br Med J II: 1511–1512
37. Creaven, PJ, Mihich, E (1977) The clinical toxicity of anticancer drugs and its prediction. Sem Oncol 4: 147–163
38. Creutzfeldt, W (1982) Proceedings of the first international symposium on acarbose. Excerpta Medica, Amsterdam
39. Creutzfeldt, W, Willms, B, Caspary, WF (1971) The mechanism of action of blood glucose lowering biguanides. In: Rodríguez RR, Vallance Owen, J (eds) Diabetes, Excerpta Medica, Amsterdam, p 95
40. Dietschy, JM, Siperstein, MD (1965) Cholesterol synthesis by the gastrointestinal tract: localisation and mechanisms of control. J Clin Invest 44: 1311–1327

41. Dimitriadis, GD, Tessari, P, Go, VLW, Gerich, JE (1985) α-Glucosidase-Hemmung bessert die postprandiale Hyperglykämie und senkt den Insulinbedarf bei insulinpflichtgem Diabetes mellitus. Dtsch Ärztebl 82: 1413–1423

42. Dixon, W, Paulley, F (1962) Anticholinergic agents favours small intestinal overgrowth during long term application. Med J Aust 3: 737–740

43. Dobbins, WO, Herrero, BA, Mansbach, CM (1968) Morphologie alterations associated with neomycin induced malabsorption. Am J Med Sci 63–77

44. Ebert, R, Bornmann, V, Creutzfeldt, W (1990) Wirkungen von Motilin und Erythromycin auf die Magenentleerung und metabolische Antwort nach Glucosegabe bei Normalpersonen. Z Gastroenterol 29: 448 (abstract)

45. Ecknaer, R (1983) Dünndarmveränderungen unter Zytostatika. In: Caspary, WF (ed) Handbuch der Inneren Medizin, Vol. III/3 B Dünndarm, Springer, Berlin Heidelberg New York, pp 571–597

46. Ehrenfeld, M, Levy, M, Sharon, P, Rachmilewitz, D, Eliakim, M (1982) Gastrointestinal effects of long-term colchicine therapy in patients with recurrent polyserositis (familial Mediterranean fever). Dig Dis Sci 27: 723–727

47. Ehrhard-Schmelzer, S, Lembcke, B, Cremer, P, Caspary, WF, Creutzfeldt, W (1983) Kontrollierte Studie über den Effekt von Guar bei ambulanten Typ-II-Diabetikern. In: Huth, K, Bräuning, C (eds) Pflanzenfasern – Neue Wege in der Stoffwechseltherapie. Beiträge zu Infusionstherapie und klinischen Ernährung – Forschung und Praxis, vol. 12. Karger, Basel, pp 195–205

48. Eichler, HG, Korn, A, Gasic, S, Pirson, W, Businger, J (1984) The effect of a new specific α-amylase inhibitor on postprandial glucose and insulin excursions in normal subjects and type 2 (noninsulin-dependent) diabetic patients. Diabetologia 26: 278–281

49. Elsenhans, B, Süfke, U, Blume, R, Caspary, WF, (1980) The influence of carbohydrate gelling agents on rat intestinal transport of monosaccharides and neutral amino acids in vitro. Clin Sci 59: 373–380

50. Elsenhans, B, Süfke, U, Blume, R, Caspary, WF (1981) In vitro inhibition of rat intestinal surface hydrolysis of disaccharides and dipeptides by guaran. Digestion 21: 98–103

51. Elsenhans, B (1983) Pharmacology of carbohydrate gelling agents. In: Creutzfeldt, W, Fölsch, UR (eds) Delaying absorption as a therapeutic principle in metabolic diseases. Thieme, Stuttgart, pp 29–43

52. Elsenhans, B, Zenker, R, Caspary, WF (1984) Guaran effect on rat intestinal absorption. A perfusion study. Gastroenterology 86: 645–653

53. Eyssen, H, Evrad, E, Vanderhaege, H (1966) Cholesterol-lowering effects of N-methylated neomycin and basic antibiotics. J Lab Clin Med 68: 753–768

54. Faloon, WW (1970) Metabolic effects of nonabsorbable antibacteria agents. Am J Clin Nutr 23: 645–651

55. Faloon, WW, Woolfolk, D, Nankin, H, Wallace, K, Haro, EN (1964) The role of bile salts in neomycin induced malabsorption. J Clin Invest 43: 1254

56. Faloon, WW, Paes, IC, Wollfolk, D, Nankin, K, Wallace, K, Haro, EN (1966) Effect of neomycin and kanamycin upon intestinal absorption. Ann New York Acad Sci 132: 879–887

57. Faloon, WW, Rublis, A, Race, TF, Webb, DI (1969) Colchicine and cholesterol metabolism. Am J Clin Nutr 22: 671–672

58. Flourie, B, Vidon, N, Florent, CH, Bernier, JJ (1984) Effect of pectin on jejunal glucose absorption and unstirred layer thickness in normal man. Gut 25: 936–941

59. Fölsch, UR, Ebert, R, Creutzfeldt, W (1981) Response of serum levels of gastric inhibitory polypeptide and insulin to sucrose ingestion during long-term application of acarbose. Scand J Gastroenterol 16: 629–632

60. Frizzel, RA, Nellans, HN, Acheson, LS (1973) Effect of cycloheximide on influx across the brush border membrane of rabbit intestine. Biochem Biophys Acta 191: 302–307

61. Garty, M, Hurtwitz, A (1980) Effect of cimetidine and antacids on gastrointestinal absorption of tetracycline. Clin Pharmacol Ther 28: 225–228
62. Gottesbühren, H, Raida, H, Riecken, EO (1974) Untersuchungen zum Einfluß von Prenylamin auf die Dünndarmresorption beim Menschen. Dtsch Med Wochenschr 99: 2104–2105
63. Gross, L, Brotman, M (1970) Hypoprothrombinemia and hemorrhage associated with cholestyramine therapy. Ann Int Med 72: 95–96
64. Gugler, R, Allgayer, H (1990) Effects of antacids on the clinical pharmacokinetics of drugs. Clin Pharmacokinet 3: 210–219
65. Gyr, K, Berger, W, Göschke, H, Stalder, GA (1970) Postprandiale Beschwerden nach Gastrektomie und ihre Beeinflussung durch Dimethylbiguanid. Dtsch Med Wochenschr 95: 2421–2431
66. Hahn, TJ, Hendin, BA, Scharp, CR (1975) Serum 25-hydroxy-cholecalciferol levels and bone mass in children on chronic anticonvulsant therapy. N Engl J Med 292: 550–554
67. Hall, GJL, Davies, AE (1969) Inhibition of iron absorption by magnesium trisilicate. Med J Aust 10: 95–96
68. Hampton, JC (1966) A comparison of the effects of irradiation and colchicine on the intestinal mucosa of the mouse. Rad Res 28: 37–59
69. Harmuth-Hoene, AE, Schelenz, R (1980) Effect of dietary fiber on mineral absorption in growing rats. J Clin Nutr 110: 1774–1784
70. Hartwich, G (1974) Side effects of a cytostatic treatment on the gastrointestinal tract. Acta Hepatogastroenterol 21: 89–92
71. Hartwich, G, Domschke, W, Matzkies, F, Pesch, HG (1975) Disaccharidases in rat small intestine mucosa following cytostatic treatment with adriamycin. Res Exp Med 166: 23–34
72. Heaton, KW, Lever, JV, Barnard, D (1972) Osteomalecia associated with cholestyramine therapy for postilectomy diarrhea. Gastroenterology 62: 642–646
73. Herbst, JJ, Hurwitz, R, Sunshine, P, Kretchmer, N (1970) Effects of colchicine on intestinal disaccharidases: corellation with biochemical aspects of cellular renewal. J Clin Invest 49: 530–536
74. Höffken, G, Lode, H, Wiley, R, Glatzel, TD, Slevers, D (1988) Pharmacokinetics and bioavailability of ciprofloxacin and ofloxacin: effect of food and antacid intake. Rec Infect Dis 20: 138–139
75. Holgate, AM, Read, NW (1983) Relationship between small bowel transit time and absorption of a solid meal. Influence of metoclopramide, magnesium sulfat, and lactulose. Dig Dis Sci 28: 812–819
76. Hollingsworth, DR, Amatruda, TT (1969) Toxic and therapeutic effects of EMTP in obesity. Clin Pharmacol Ther 10: 540–542
77. Houlihan, M, Scott, JM, Boyle, PH, Wier, DB (1972) The effect of phenytoin on the absorption of synthetic folic acid polyglutamate. Gut 13: 189–190
78. Hvidt, S, Kjeldsen, K (1963) Malabsorption induced by small doses of neomycin sulfate. Acta Med Scand 173: 699 (abstract)
79. Insogna, KL, Bordly, DR, Card, RJ, Lockwood, DA (1980) Osteomalacia and weakness. In: Jacobson, ED, Prior, JT, Faloon, WW (1960) Malabsorptive syndrome induced by neomycin: morphologic alterations in the jejunal mucosa. J Lab Clin Med 56: 245–250
80. Jacobson, ED, Chodos, RB, Faloon, WW (1960) An experimental malabsorption syndrome induced by neomycin. Am J Med 28: 524–533
81. Janssens, J, Peeters, TL, Vantrappen, G, Tack, J, Urbain, JL, DeRoo, M, Muls, E, Boulllion, R (1990) Improvement of gastric emptying in diabetic gastroparesis by erythromycin: preliminary studies. N Engl J Med 322: 1028–1030
82. Jenkins, DJA, Leeds, AR, Slavin, B, Mann, J, Jepson, EM (1979) Dietary fiber and blood lipids: reduction of serum cholesterol in type II hyperlipidemia by guar gum. Am J Clin Nutr 32: 16–18

83. Jenkins, DJA, Hill, MS, Cummings, JH (1975) Effect of wheat fiber on blood lipids, fecal steroid excretion and serum iron. Am J Clin Nutr 28: 1408–1411

84. Layer, P, Carlson, GL, DiMagno, EP (1985) Partially purified white bean amylase inhibitor reduces starch digestion in vitro and inactivates intraduodenal amylase in humanes. Gastroenterology 88: 1895–1902

85. Lembcke, B, Caspary, WF (1977) Dipeptid-Transport-Beeinflussung durch Phenformin. Z Gastroenterol 15: [suppl] 36–38

86. Lembcke, B (1987) Beeinflussung der Resorption – Resorptionsverzögerung als therapeutisches Prinzip. In: Caspary, WF (ed) Diabetes Forum I: Struktur und Funktion des Dünndarmes – Therapie des Diabetes mellitus. Excerpta Medica, Amsterdam, pp 269–287

87. Lembcke, B, Caspary, WF (1983) Atemanalytische Funktionstests. In: Caspary, WF (ed) Handbuch der Inneren Medizin, vol. III/3 A Dünndarm, Springer, Berlin, Heidelberg, New York, pp 488–520

88. Lembcke, B, Caspary, WF (1988) Malabsorption syndromes. Clin Gastroenterol 2: 329–351

89. Lembcke, B, Creutzfeldt, W, Schleser, S, Ebert, R, Shaw, C, Koop, I (1987) Effect of somatostatin analogue sandostatin (SMS 201–995) on gastrointestinal, pancreatic and biliary function and hormone release in normal man. Digestion 36: 108–124

90. Lembcke, B, Diederich, M, Fölsch, UR, Creutzfeldt (1990) Postprandial glycemic control, hormonal effects and carbohydrate malabsorption during long-term administration of the α-glucosidase inhibitor miglitol. Digestion 47: 47–55

91. Lembcke, B, Fuchs, C, Hesch, RD, Caspary, WF (1982) Effect of long term antacid administration on mineral metabolism. In: Halter, F (ed) Antacids in the eighties, Urban Schwarzenberg, Munich, pp 112–122

92. Leveille, GA, Powel, RC, Sauberlich, HE, Nunes, WT (1963) Effect of orally and parenterally administered neomycin on plasma lipids in normal subjects. Am J Clin Nutr 12: 421–426

93. Levin, RJ (1968) Anatomical and functional changes on the small intestine induced by 5-fluorouracil. J Physiol 197: 73–74

94. Lotz, M, Zisman, E, Bartter, FC (1968) Evidence of a phosphorus depletion syndrome in man. N Engl J Med 278: 409–415

95. MacKenzie, IJ, Donaldson, RM (1972) Effect of divalent kations and pH on intrinsic factor-mediated attachment of vitamin B_{12} to intestinal microvillous membranes. J Clin Invest 51: 2465–2471

96. Mantylä, R, Männisto, PT, Vuorela, A, Sunderberg, S, Ottoila, P (1984) Impairment of captopril bioavailability by concomitant food and antacid intake. Int J Clin Pharmacol Ther Toxicol 33: 626–629

97. Maxwell, JD, Hunter, J, Stewart, DA, Ardeman, S, Williams, R (1972) Folate deficiency after anticonvulsant drugs: an effect of hepatic enzyme induction? Br Med J 1: 297–299

98. Meyer, BH, Müller, FO, Clur, BK, Grigoleit, HG (1983) Effects of tendamistate (α-amylase inactivator) on starch metabolism. Br J Clin Pharmacol 16: 145–148

99. Mizuno, M, Hamaura, T, Hashida, M, Sezaki, H (1986) Changes in D-glucose uptake by brush border vesicles from small intestine of rats treated with mitomycin C. Biochem Pharmacol 35: 1153–1158

100. Olsen, WA, Rasmussen, HK (1974) Effect of phenformin on carbohydrate absorption in man. Diabetes 23: 716–718

101. Paes, IC, Searl, B, Rubert, MW, Faloon, WW (1967) Intestinal lactase deficiency and saccharidase malabsorption during oral neomycin administration. Gastroenterology 53: 49–58

102. Palva, IP, Salokannel, SJ, Timonen, T, Myränen, J (1972) Malabsorption and deficiency of vitamin B_{12} during treatment with slow-release potassium chloride. Acta Med Scand 191: 355–357

103. Pinkerton, CR, Milla, JP (1984) Methotrexate enterotoxicity: Influence of drug dose and timing in the rat. Br J Cancer 49: 97–101
104. Ponz de Leon, M, Iori, R, Barbolini, G, Pompei, G, Zaniol, P, Carulli, N (1982) Influence of small bowel transit time on dietary cholesterol absorption in human beings. N Engl J Med 307: 102–103
105. Puls, W, Krause, HP, Müller, L, Schutt, H, Sitt, R, Thomas, G (1984) Inhibitors on the rate of carbohydrate and lipid absorption by the intestine. Int J Obesity 8: (suppl. 1) 181–190
106. Race, TF, Paes, IC, Faloon, WW (1970) Intestinal malabsorption induced by oral colchicine. Comparison with neomycin and carthartic agents. Am J Med Sci 259: 32–41
107. Reinhold, JG, Nasr, K, Lahimgarzadeh, A, Hedayatti, H (1973) Effects of purified phytate and phytate rich bread upon metabolism of zinc, calcium, phosphorus and nitrogen in man. Lancet I: 283–288
108. Reisenauer, AM, Halsted, CH (1981) Human jejunal brush border folate conjugase. Characteristics and inhibition by salicylasulfapyridine. Biochim Biophys Acta 659: 62–69
109. Riecken, EO, Rosenbaum, R, Bloch, R, Creutzfeldt, W (1969) Tierexperimentelle Untersuchungen zur Frage der Spezifität der Dünndarmschleimhautveränderungen bei der einheimischen Sprue. Klin Wochenschr 47: 202–214
110. Robinson, JWL (1972) Experimental intestinal malabsorption states and their relation to clinical syndromes. Klin Wochenschr 50: 173–185
111. Robinson, JWL, Antoniolo, JA, Vannotti, A (1966) The effect of oral methotrexate on the rat intestine. Biochem Pharmacol 15: 1479–1489
112. Roche, AC, Bognel, JCL, Bognel, C, Bernier, JJ (1970) Correlation between the histological changes and glucose intestinal absorption following a single dose of 5-fluorouracil. Digestion 3: 195–212
113. Rosenberg, IH (1981) Intestinal absorption of folate. In: Johnson, LR, Christensen, J, Grossman, MI, Jacobson, ED, Schultz, SG (eds) Physiology of the gastrointestinal tract, vol. 2. Raven, New York, pp 1221–1230
114. Rosenberg, IH, Godwin, HA, Streiff, RR, Castle, WB (1968) Impairment of intestinal deconjugation of dietary folate: a possible explanation of megaloblastic anemia associated with phenytoin therapy. Lancet II: 530–532
115. Rublis, A, Rubert, M, Faloon, WW (1970) Cholesterol lowering, fecal bile acid, and sterol changes during neomycin and colchicine. Am J Clin Nutr 28: 1251–1259
116. Sarna, SK, Soergel, KH, Koch, TR, Stone, JE, Wood, CM, Ryan, RP, Arndorfer, RC, Cavanaugh, JH, Nellans, HN, Lee, MB (1991) Gastrointestinal motor effects of erythromycin in humans. Gastroenterology 101: 1488–1496
117. Samuel, P, Salchi, OB, Holtzman, CM (1964) Reduction of serum cholesterol concentrations by paromomycin in patients with atherosclerosis. Proc Soc Exp Biol Med 115: 718–721
118. Sedahagat, A, Samuel, P, Crouse, JR, Ahrens, EH (1975) Effect of neomycin on absorption, synthesis, and/or flux of cholesterol in man. J Clin Invest 55: 12–21
119. Shelly, DW, Doering, PL, Russel, WL, Guild, RT, López, LM (1986) Effect of concomitant antacid administration on plasma cimetidine concentrations during repetitive dosing. Drug Intell Clin Pharm 20: 792–795
120. Shields, HM (1978) Rapid fall of serum phosphorus secondary to antacid therapy. Gastroenterology 75: 1137–1141
121. Spencer, H, Lender, M (1979) Adverse effects of aluminium-containing antacids on mineral metabolism. Gastroenterology 76: 603–606
122. Steinberg, WM, Lewis, JH, Katz, DM (1982) Antacids inhibit absorption of cimetidine. N Engl J Med 307: 400–404
123. Steiner, A, Howard, E, Akgun, S (1961) Effect of antibiotics on the serum cholesterol concentration of patients with atherosclerosis. Circulation 24: 729–735

124. Stemmerman, GN, Hayashi, T (1971) Colchicine intoxication: a reappraisal of its pathology based on a study of three fatal cases. Hum Pathol 2: 321–328

125. Szatloczky, E (1971) Behandlung des Dumping-Syndromes mit zuckerresorptionshemmenden Mitteln. Dtsch Med Wochenschr 96: 308–311

126. Thomas, FB, Salsburey, D, Greenberger, NJ (1972) Inhibition of iron absorption by cholestyramine: demonstration of diminished iron stores following prolonged administration. Am J Dig Dis Sci 17: 263–269

127. Thompson, GR, Barrowman, J, Gutiérrez, L, Dowling, H (1971) Action of neomycin on the intraluminal phase of lipid absorption. J Clin Invest 50: 319–323

128. Tomkin, GH (1973) Malabsorption of vitamin B_{12} in diabetic patients treated with phenformin. A comparison with metformin. Br Med J 3: 673–675

129. Trier, JS (1962) Morphologic alterations induced by methotraxate in the mucosa of human proximal intestine. I. Serial observations by light microscopy. Gastroenterology 42: 295–309

130. Trier, JS (1962) Morphologic alterations induced by methotrexate in the mucosa of human proximal intestine. II. Electron microscopy observations. Gastroenterology 43: 407–423

131. Vince, A, Killingley, M, Wrong, OM (1978) Effect of lactulose on ammonia production in a fecal incubation system. Gastroenterology 74: 544–549

132. West, JR, Lloyd, JK (1975) The effect of cholestyramine on intestinal absorption. GUT 16: 93–98

133. Zimmerman, JR, Selhub, J, Rosenberg, IH (1985) Drug-folate interactions in intestinal folate absorption: comparison of sulfasalazine, phenytoin, and salicylates. Gastroenterology 88: 1643–1646

Disturbance of the Intestinal Ecosystem by Antimicrobial Agents

P. C. Braga

Department of Pharmacology, School of Medicine, University of Milan

1 Introduction

Antibiotics are the most widely used class of drugs and differ from other pharmacological agents commonly used for therapy in that their action is addressed to cells not belonging to human body, for example, bacteria, while other drugs acts on cells of the human body. This means that among the huge number of substances with antimicrobial activity, only those that have specific affinity for micro-organisms and not for human cells are chosen for therapy.

Since the pathogens are in contact with the inside of our bodies, to act on pathogens antimicrobial drugs must also be in contact with the cells of our bodies. Although they have been chosen for their selectivity, antibiotics can also cause side effects. It is frequently forgotten in medicine that human organisms harbor ample microbial flora, almost entirely concentrated in the intestine and forming an integral part of the human body. Intestinal microflora reaches $10^{10}-10^{13}$ bacteria per gram of feces (dry weight), but the most striking fact is that the total number of bacteria present in the human intestine is about equal to the total number of cells of the human body [70].

In normal conditions this enormous number of bacteria (about 400 or more bacterial species can be identified [24]) is distributed along the human intestine according to their possibilities of colonization (Fig. 1). The virtual "absence" of oxygen in the intestine creates a favorable environment for anaerobic enteric microflora.

Enteric microflora has complex metabolic activities that influence the human host, and the physiological homeostasis between the host and its intestinal microflora generally results in reciprocal benefit (Table 1).

Table 1. Functions exerted by enteric microflora on the host animal

Action on	
● Intestine	Morphology, function, motility
● Digestive processes	Fermentative flora (ascending colon) digests starch; putrefactive flora (left colon) digests proteins
● Metabolism	Biliary acid, steroid hormones (estrogens/androgens), drugs, xenobiotics
Production of	
● Intestinal gas	Volume, composition
● Vitamins	K, B complex
● Metabolites	Toxic, carcinogens/mutagens
Control of	
● Feces	Composition, characteristics
● Regional bioelectric potential	pH, ox-redox potential

Infections are automatically treated with antibiotics to kill the offending micro-organism, but when antibiotics enter the human body, their distribution cannot be oriented exclusively to the tissue or organ invaded by bacteria. Thus, large or small amounts of antibiotic also reach the intes-

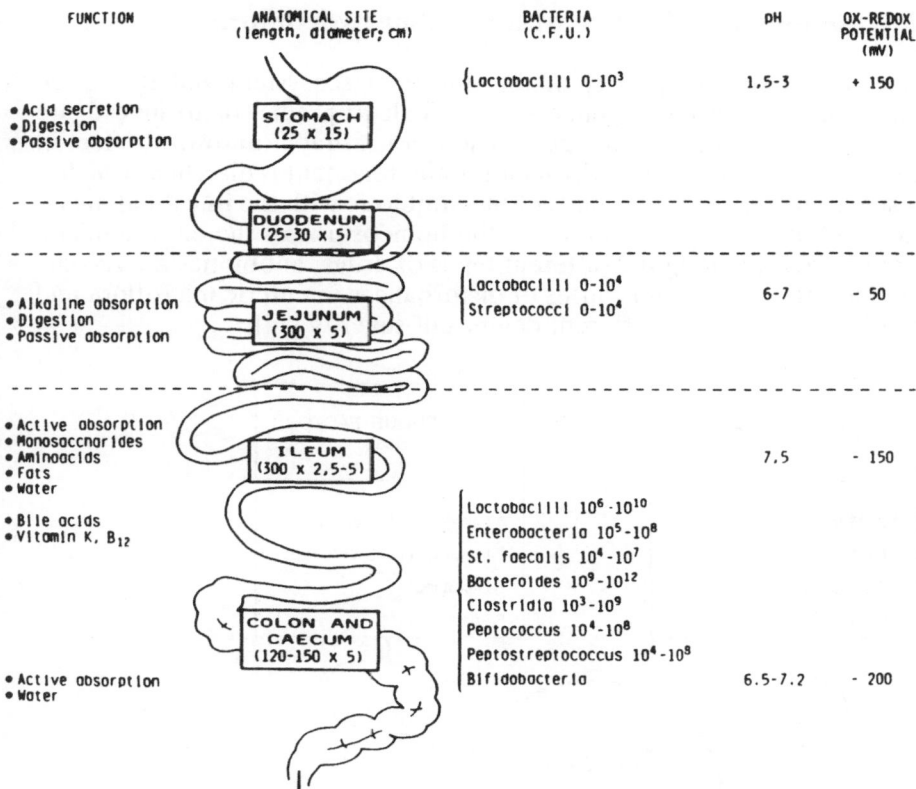

FUNCTION	ANATOMICAL SITE (length, diameter; cm)	BACTERIA (C.F.U.)	pH	OX-REDOX POTENTIAL (mV)
• Acid secretion • Digestion • Passive absorption	STOMACH (25 x 15)	{Lactobacilli 0-10³	1,5-3	+ 150
• Alkaline absorption • Digestion • Passive absorption	DUODENUM (25-30 x 5) JEJUNUM (300 x 5)	{Lactobacilli 0-10⁴ Streptococci 0-10⁴	6-7	- 50
• Active absorption • Monosaccharides • Aminoacids • Fats • Water • Bile acids • Vitamin K, B₁₂	ILEUM (300 x 2,5-5)		7,5	- 150
• Active absorption • Water	COLON AND CAECUM (120-150 x 5)	Lactobacilli 10⁶ -10¹⁰ Enterobacteria 10⁵-10⁸ St. faecalis 10⁴-10⁷ Bacteroides 10⁹-10¹² Clostridia 10³-10⁹ Peptococcus 10⁴-10⁸ Peptostreptococcus 10⁴-10⁸ Bifidobacteria	6.5-7.2	- 200

Fig. 1. Schematic outline of intestinal structure, function, pH, ox-redox ptential and regional distribution of bacteria in the human intestine. (With permission from [4])

tine (depending on the route of administration – oral, parenteral, etc.) and therefore also act on the saprophytic enteric microflora.

Many different parameters play a role in the balance between the intestinal ecosystem and antibiotics. Because of their specific mechanisms of action some of these affect not only the pathogenic bacteria but also the useful saprophytic bacteria and can disrupt the equilibrium between different resident species, some of which decrease in number and in distribution while others increase in number and can colonize an unoccupied habitat [71]. The nature and degree of this interaction and of the new equilibrium, which can be detrimental to the human host, depends on the previous composition of the flora, the spectrum of activity and dose and duration of administration of the antibiotic.

2 Antibiotic Interference with Intestinal Microflora

Because of the complexity of the intestinal ecosystem and the differences in antimicrobial agents, it is difficult to predict or to investigate
the exact effect of a given agent. The most frequent untoward effect in
the intestine associated with an antibiotic treatment is diarrhea, which is
a sign of negative interference of the antibiotic with the intestinal microflora. Many factors can influence the homeostasis of the enteric microflora (Fig. 2); among the different types of drugs, antibiotics are recognized as one of the main causes of disturbances in enteric microflora and
intestinal diseases of different degrees of severity [14].

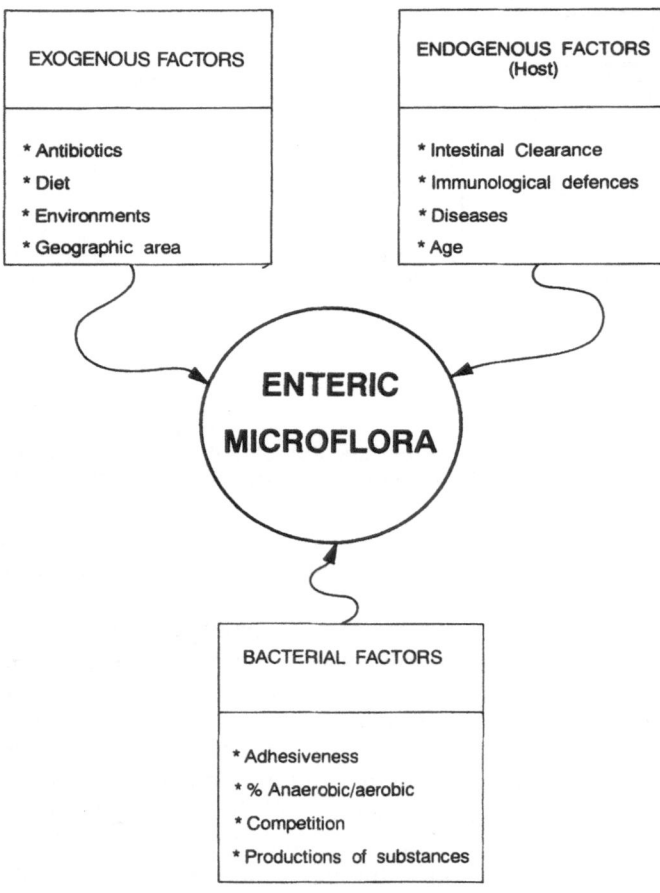

Fig. 2. Main factors influencing enteric microflora

2.1 Simple Diarrhea

If gastrointestinal symptoms such as vomiting and diarrhea occur immediately (one or few hours) after antibiotic ingestion, they are usually due to a direct toxic side effect, which is uncommon with antibiotics. Generally when there is only diarrhea, not immediately but after several administrations of antibiotic, this is attributable to interference with the enteric microflora, with changes in regional colonization, with the predominance of local strains that produce different kinds of toxins, which in turn induce initial dysfunction in fluid absorption and electrolyte transport by the villi, changes in osmolality, in villi morphology and successive villi damage, and edema of the lamina propria [75].

The diarrhea ascribed to antibiotics generally consists of relatively large volume loose or watery stools, sometimes with mucus but rarely with grossly evident blood. It may be dose related and generally resolves promptly when the antibiotic is discontinued [6, 68].

In general, the specific effects of an antimicrobial agent depend on several parameters: its spectrum of activity, the dosage, the route of administration and the concentration of active drug in the lumen of the intestine [68].

This simple diarrhea or antibiotic-associated colitis has been reported to affect 5 %–35 % of patients treated with antibiotics [6]. About 20 % of antibiotic-associated diarrheas are caused by *Clostridium difficile* [85], and this is the most severe form of antibiotic enterocolitis, also called pseudomembranous enterocolitis (PMC).

2.2 Pseudomembranous Enterocolitis

PMC was known already before there were antimicrobial drugs, and a variety of risk factors were noted (intestinal obstruction and ischemia, intestinal surgery, debilitating disease, cytotoxic therapy, low birth weight in the new born [7, 23, 44, 86], but the majority of cases currently encountered are antibiotic associated.

Up to the 1970s there was some evidence that the etiologic agent for PMC was *Staphylococcus aureus*, but in 1977 it was observed in the stools of patients with PMC a particular toxin with a cytotoxic effect and the ability to neutralize its effect by giving an antitoxin from *C. sordelli*. It was then confirmed that the toxin was produced by *C. difficile*, a gram-positive anaerobic, sporogenic bacillus. The onset of diarrhea is generally 4–10 days after the beginning of antibiotic treatment, occasionally within 3–4 weeks after cessation of antibiotic treatment. There are three to ten stools per day, which are semisolid or liquid in character; mucus or blood is seldom present. Many individuals experience nausea, vomiting, abdominal cramps, and tenderness. Fever is usually low grade; peripheral leukocyte counts are variable, 10,000–40,000 or higher [52, 79]. The diarrhea lasts on average 10–12 days.

For exact diagnosis, endoscopy is required. The distal colon is involved in the majority of cases, so that sigmoidoscopy is generally adequate. Occasionally patients have pseudomembranes restricted to the right colon, necessitating colonoscopy [77]. Radiological findings may be helpful in establishing the diagnosis of PMC [74].

The usual finding during macroscopic inspection are multiple elevated yellowish-white plaques which vary in size from a few millimeters to 12–20 mm in diameter. The surrounding mucosa may appear normal or be hyperemic and edematous. Occasionally the pseudomembranes coalesce to involve large segments of the colonic mucosa. These may slough off, leaving large denuded areas. The pseudomembrane is composed of fibrin, mucin, sloughed epithelial mucosal cells and inflammatory cells. There is an acute or chronic inflammatory infiltrate in the lamina propria, with the submucosa edematous and with vascular dilatation.

Nearly all antimicrobial agents have been implicated in both diarrhea and PCM. Exceptions are vancomycin and some parenterally administered aminoglycosides.

The first observations were described in connection with tetracyclines and chloramphenicol, but these were followed by ampicillin [19, 62], amoxycillin [72], cotrimoxazole [19], cephalosporins [27, 82], kanamycin and gentamycin [44], metronidazole [67] and more recently clindamycin and lincomycin [66, 76, 78]. The frequency of diarrhea with the latter two antibiotics can be as high as 20 % of patients treated [32].

3 Interactions of Different Classes of Antibiotics on Enteric Microflora

Figure 3 presents a flow-chart of the different steps by which antibiotics that act on enteric saprophytic strains start a cascade of events leading to the occurrence of simple diarrhea or more severe disorders such as PMC. Tables 2 and 3 compares the risks of diarrhea for different antibiotics.

3.1 β-Lactam Antibiotics

Benzylpenicillin and phenoxymethylpenicillin have narrow spectra of activity, are attacked by β-lactamase, and small amounts can be detected in the feces [29, 36, 55]. This is probably why they have little effect on enteric flora. However, phenoxymethylpenicillin has been incriminated for diarrhea and colitis caused by *C. difficile* [4].

Table 2. Comparative behavior of different antibiotics in relationship to the risk of diarrhea and to related parameters

	Spectrum	Interference of aerobes	Interference of anaerobes	Diarrhea risk	Absorption	Biliary excretion	Fecal levels	Risk of resistance	Risk of super infection
Benzylpenicillin	O	O	O	■	●●	O	O	O	O
Ampicillin	●●	●	●	■■	●●	O	●●	●	●●
Bacampicillin	●●	O	O	■	●●●	O	●	O	O
Piperacillin	●●●	●●	●●	■■	O	●	●●	●	?
Azlocillin	●●●	●●	●●	■■	O	●	●●	●	●●
Cefoperaxone	●●	●●●	●●●	■■	O	●●	●●●	●●	●●●
Ceftriaxone	●●	●●●	●●●	■■■	O	●●	●●	●●	●●●
Cefoxitin	●●●	●●●	●●●	■■	O	●	●●	●	●●
Aztreonam	O	O	O	■	O	●	●●	●	●●
Imipenem	●●●	O	O	■	O	●	●	O	?
Doxycycline	●●●	●●●	●●●	■	●●	●●	●●	●●●	●●●
Erythromycin	O	●●●	●●●	■	●●	●●	●●●	●●●	●●●
Clindamycin	O	●●	●●●	■■	●●●	●●	●●	●●	●
Norfloxacin	●●	O	O	O	●●●	●	●●	O	O
Ciprofloxacin	●●	O	O	O	●●●	●	●●	O	O
Aminoglycosides	O	●●	O	■	O	●	●	●	●
Metronidazole	O	O	O	O	●●●	●	O	O	●
Tinidazole	O	O	O	O	●●●	●	O	O	●

O, Low; ●/■, Moderate; ●●/■■, High; ●●●/■■■, Very high

Table 3. Rate of diarrhea due to therapy with antibacterial agents (from [88])

Antibacterial agent	Diarrhea among patients receiving the drug (%)	Drug excretion in bile (%)
Ampicillin	10	<1
Phenoxymethylpenicillin, benzylpenicillin	5	<1
Cloxacillin	15	5
Carbenicillin	8	2
Cefaclor	5	4
Cephalothin	4	2
Cephalexin	11	<5
Ceftriaxone	28	30
Cefoperazone	24	70
Cefoxitin	<2	<2
Ceftazidime	<2	<1
Tetracyclines	15	>10
Doxycycline	12	4–20
Chloramphenicol	7	<5
Gentamicin	4	<1
Kanamycin	4	<1
Erythromycin orally (not microencapsulated)	22	<5
Erythromycin estolate	17	–
Clindamycin/lincomycin	21	10
Sulfonamides	8	<1
Cotrimoxazole	10	<1
Nitrofurantoin	12	–
Nalidixic acid	7	–
Ciprofloxacin	<2	<1
Norfloxacin	<2	<1
Ofloxacin	<2	<1
Rifampicin	11	25

Ampicillin and its esters [46] reduce the counts of gram-positive aerobes and anaerobes and of *Bacteroides* spp. [73], and there is rather high incidence of diarrhea during treatment [31].

Piperacillin and azlocillin are excreted in high concentrations in the bile, and they markedly reduce both aerobic flora (enterococci, streptococci, enterobacteria) and anaerobic flora (cocci, nonsporulating and sporulating gram-positive rods and *Bacteroides*) [41, 57]. The same is true for ampicillin/sulbactam [39].

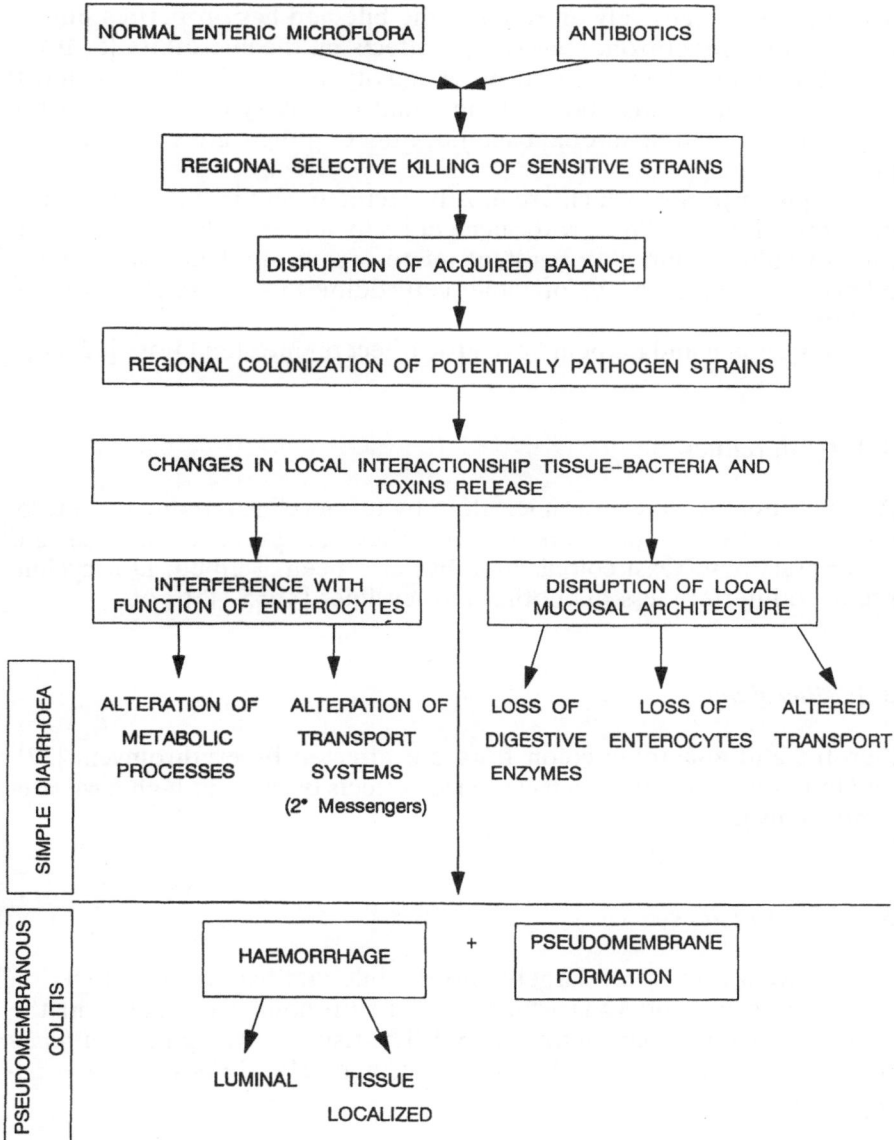

Fig. 3. Schematic flow-chart of the possible steps by which antibiotics can initiate a cascade of events leading to a disruption of the intestinal function

Cefoperazone has a broad spectrum of activity and very high concentrations in the feces are consistent with the fact that up to 75 % of a dose is eliminated in the bile [54]. These pharmacological properties greatly affect the equilibrium of the normal microflora. Ceftriaxone, which is also extensively excreted in the bile and has properties similar to those of cefoperazone, has similar effects on the microflora [5, 10].

Cefoxitin has a wide spectrum of activity and is present in the intestine in concentrations above the minimal inhibitory concentration for many aerobic and anaerobic bacteria, affecting their grow and balance [40].

Cephalosporins, which are mostly excreted via the bile, can greatly interfere with fecal flora, with such generally undesirable results as diarrhea or colonization with resistant micro-organisms. Those with minor biliary excretion (e.g., cefotaxime, ceftazidime) have less effect on microflora [63].

Aztreonam and imipem have little effect on intestinal flora [42, 56].

3.2 Tetracyclines

A great effect is shown on microflora by tetracyclines, reducing enterococci and other aerobic streptococci; they can produce diarrhea and superinfections. Yeast colonization has also been ascribed. Doxicycline seems to interfere less than other tetracyclines [4, 35, 45].

3.3 Macrolides

Aerobic and anaerobic colon flora are affected by erythromycin [37], and long-term treatment can cause side effects because of high fecal concentrations [58].

3.4 Lincosamides

Clindamycin is excreted largely into the bile and has strong activity on anaerobic cocci and rods which leads to pronounced changes in the aerobic and anaerobic microflora [55]. The risk of developing *C. difficile* diarrhea is well established and can occur in 2% – 20% of treated patients [35, 48].

3.5 Quinolones

Older quinolones (e.g., nalidixic acid) do not affect enterobacteriaceae significantly [83], while the newer fluorinated quinolones affect both gram-positive and gram-negative bacteria, especially Enterobacteriaceae. Their activities against anaerobic bacteria are limited [26], and no significant effects on the fecal flora have been reported [63].

3.6 Aminoglycosides

Parenterally administered aminoglycosides are generally excreted very little into the bile and thus have little effect on the fecal flora [30]. Orally administered aminoglycosides tend to interfere with the aerobic flora and gram-positive anaerobes [69, 87].

3.7 Cotrimoxazole

A similar effect is seen on the enteric flora with cotrimoxazole as with quinolones: suppression of Enterobacteriaceae, while anaerobic flora is unaffected [84]. However, PMC has been observed, although less frequently than with other antibacterial drugs [19].

3.8 Imidazole Derivatives

Metronidazole, ornidazole, tinidazole, are active at therapeutic doses against anaerobic microorganisms. Aerobes and enterococci are not affected [16, 17, 30, 38].

3.9 Chloramphenicol, Thiamphenicol

Dose-dependent gastrointestinal disturbances are diarrhea, nausea, or constipation and occur in fewer than 10 % of cases but are usually mild [25].

3.10 Rifampicin

Diarrhea and pseudomembranous colitis can be induced by rifampicin [25, 28].

4 Malabsorption Induced by Antibiotics

Among the different causes of malabsorption, the antibiotic-induced unbalance in enteric microflora can also both induce defects of absorption and negatively interfere with the complex metabolic activities of a well-balanced microflora, for instance the production of vitamin K and the B complex [13]. Administration of antibiotics has been associated with impaired absorption of a variety of therapeutic agents, even when there is no diarrhea of steatorrhea [9, 22].

Bacterial enzymes also include β-glucuronidases, sulfatases, and various glycosidases. Antibiotics interfering with intestinal bacteria also alter the amount and distribution of these enzymes. Many drugs and endogenous compounds, such as estrogens, folic acid, bile acids, cholesterol, ouabain, digoxin, promazine, morphine, diethylstilbestrol, etc. have an enterohepatic recycle and are generally conjugated to a polar group such as glucuronic acid, sulfate, taurine, glycine, or glutathione prior to secretion in the bile. The low level of bacterial hydrolizing enzymes cannot completely deconjugate these agents, and they can be reabsorbed with unpredictable effects [13, 49, 50, 64] (see also Chap. 7, this volume).

5 Treatment

When there is antibiotic-associated diarrhea, colitis or PMC, the first therapeutic approach consists of stopping the antibiotic and giving fluid and electrolytes because with diarrhea fluid losses can reach 10–15 l per day, and serum proteins and in some cases blood are also lost. These must be replaced with plasma, albumin, or blood transfusions. Since the etiologic agent is a bacterium (*C. difficile*), the adopted therapy is antibacterial therapy; thus there is a curious circle the "iatrogenic" pathology induced by antibiotics is treated with other antibiotics.

5.1 Vancomycin

If the cause is a toxin-producing *Clostridium,* oral vancomycin is at present the most effective form of treatment [33, 80]. Daily doses from 500 mg to 2 g vancomycin for 7 days is the most common adopted therapy, which promptly eradicates fever within 24–48 h in 80 % of patients, and diarrhea is resolved on average in 4,5 days (range 1–13 days) [8]. The only problem is that 19 % of patients develop relapses after discontinuation of vancomycin [8]. After a second course of vancomycin, about 20 %–30 % of these patients suffer another relapse [8]. This probably means that there are still spores of *C. difficile,* and vancomycin is not active against spores.

5.2 Teicoplanin

This is a glicopeptide antibiotic structurally related to vancomycin. The antibacterial activity of teicoplanin, as that of vancomycin, is restricted to gram-positive aerobic and anaerobic micro-organisms. Teicoplanin has some advantages over vancomycin: it has a longer elimination half-life so that it can be administered every 24 h, it can also be administered intramuscularly, and it has greater degree of antibacterial activity [47]. Teicoplanin is about two to four times more active than vancomycin against *C. difficile* and other *Clostridium* spp. [34, 53, 60], and it may prove useful for the same indication as for vancomycin.

5.3 Rifaximin

A new derivative of rifamycin SV, rifaximin can be administered orally but is not absorbed by intestinal tract and is not inactivated by low pH of the stomach [2]. Its spectrum of activity cover both gram-positive and gram-negative intestinal aerobic and anaerobic flora [65]. Rifaximin is also active in pseudomembranous colitis caused by *C. difficile;* it was more effective than neomycin but less effective than vancomycin [11, 65].

5.4 Anion Exchange Resins

Cholestyramine binds the toxin produced by *C. difficile* [18, 20], which is the rationale for its use in PMC. A dose of 4 g three times a day for 5 days results in prompt improvement of symptoms, with the only side effect being constipation. However, results are variable.

5.5 Vamcomycin plus Cholestyramine

To try to improve clinical results, concurrent administration of vancomycin plus cholestyramine has been proposed. However, the anion-binding resin also binds vancomycin, thus lowering biologically active levels of this drug.

5.6 Bacitracin

This agent is active in vitro against *C. difficile* [21] and is poorly absorbed when administered orally; thus intestinal concentrations are high. The reported experience with this drug is limited, but results appear promising.

5.7 Metronidazole

An extremely active agent against anaerobic bacteria and *C. difficile* is metronidazole. However, it is well absorbed so that intestinal concentrations are low [3]. Even with this disadvantage some favorable results have appeared in the literature [51, 59, 61], although this drug has also been implicated as causal agent in at least nine cases of PMC with positive toxin assays [43, 67, 81].

5.8 Antitoxin

The toxin from *C. difficile* can be neutralized by antitoxin to *C. difficile* or *C. sordelli*. This might be effective therapeutically, as shown in experimental animals after intraluminal injections (laparatomy) [1].

5.9 Manipulation of the Fecal Flora

PMC mediated by the *C. difficile* toxin requires both the presence of *C. difficile* and antibiotic exposure. This is because the competing flora are reduced by antibiotic, and *C. difficile* can colonize part of the intestine. There is a report that fecal enemas gives good results in 13 of 16 patients [12] so that the possibility of reestablishing normal flora or competing flora to inhibit *C. difficile* should be considered. Table 4 reports other possible ways to act on intestinal dysbiosis by administration of the micro-organisms used in oral bacteriotherapy [15].

Table 4. Factors inducing changes in the enteric microflora

Type of preparation	Microorganisms
Microorganisms not belonging to enteric flora (oral administration)	*Saccharomyces boulardii* *Saccharomyces cerevisiae* *Bacillus subtilis*
Microorganisms belonging to enteric flora (oral administration)	Lactobacilli *Bifidobacterium bifidus* *Enterococcus faecium*
Mixture of purified bacterial antigen fractions (oral administration)	*Escherichia coli* *Enterococcus faecalis* *Stafilococcus aureus* *Proteus vulgaris* *Proteus morgagni* *Bacillus subtilis* *Bacillus mesentericus* *Bacillus faecalis* *Aerobacter aerogens*
Oral vaccines	*Escherichia coli* (lysates)

5.10 Antidiarrheal Drugs

The use of antidiarrhea drugs for symptomatic relief must be avoided because they favor persistence of toxin in the intestinal lumen.

6 Conclusions

The need to use antibiotics to treat infections can be detrimental to the useful saprophitic intestinal microflora. The resulting clinical situation can be a simple, generally self-limiting diarrhea, but a pseudomembranous colitis, induced by toxins from *C. difficile,* can also arise. This situation can have potentially severe consequences also in relationship with the degree of electrolites and proteins losses. The recognized therapy with vancomycin given orally at present shows the most rapid and best clinical results.

References

1. Allo, M, Salva, J Jr, Fekety, R et al. (1979) Prevention of clindamycin-induced colitis in hamsters by Clostridia sordelli antitoxin. Gastroenterology 76: 351–355
2. Alvisi, V, D'Ambrosi, A, Loponte, A, Pazzi, P, Greco, A, Zangirolami, A, Palazzini, E (1987) Rifaximin, a rifamycin derivative for the use in the treatment of intestinal bacterial infections in seriously disabled patients. J Int Med Res 15: 59–56
3. Arabi, T, Dimock, F, Burdon, DW et al. (1979) Influence of neomycin and metronidazole on colonic microflora of volunteers. J Antimicrob Chemother 5: 531–537
4. Aronsson, B, Möllby, R, Nord, CE (1985) Antimicrobial agents and Clostridium difficile in acute enteric disease: epidemiological data from Sweden 1980/82. J Infect Dis 151: 476–481
5. Arvidsson, A, Alvan, G, Angelin, B, Borga, O, Nord, CE (1982) Ceftriaxone: renal and biliary excretion and effect on the colon microflora. J Antimicr Chemother 10: 207–215
6. Ashkenazi, S, Cleary, TG, Pickering, LK (1989) Bacterial toxins associated with diarrheal disease. In: Lebenthal, E, Duffey, M (eds) Textbook of secretory diarrhea. Raven, New York
7. Bartlett, JG, Gorbach, SL (1977) Pseudomembranous enterocolitis (antibiotic-related colitis). Ad Intern Med 22: 455–460
8. Bartlett, JG, Tedesco, FJ, Shull, S, Lowe, B (1979) Symptomatic relaps after oral vancomycin therapy of antibiotic-associated pseudomembranous colitis. Gastroenterology 78: 431–434
8a. Bergan, T (1986) Pharmacokinetic differentiation and consequences for normal microflora. Scand J Infect Dis 49 (Suppl): 91–99
9. Bint, AJ, Burtt, I (1980) Adverse antibiotic drug interaction. Drugs 20: 57–69
10. Bodey, GP, Fainstein, V, Garcìa, I, Rosenbaum, B, Wong, Y (1983) Effect of broad-spectrum cephalosporins on the microbial flora of recipients. J Infect Dis 148: 892–897
11. Boero, M, Berti, E, Morgando, A, Verme, G (1990) Terapia della colite da Clostridium difficile: risultati di uno studio randomizzato aperto rifaximina vs. vancomicina. Microbiol Medica 5: 74–77

12. Bowden, TA, Jr, Mausberger, AR, Jr, Lykins, LE (1981) Pseumomembranous enterocolitis: mechanism for restoring floral homeostasis. Am Surg 47: 178–184

13. Braga, PC (1991) Interaction of antibiotics on enteric microflora. In Braga, PC, Guslandi, M, Tittobello, A (eds) Drugs in gastroenterology. Raven, New York, pp 509–517

14. Braga, PC (1991) Enteric microflora and its regulation. In: Braga PC, Guslandi M, Tittobello A (eds) Drugs in gastroenterology. Raven, New York, pp 501–507

15. Braga, PC (1991) Microorganisms regulating enteric microflora. In: Braga, PC, Guslandi, M, Tittobello, A (eds) Drugs in gastroenterology. Raven, New York, pp 518–523

16. Braga, PC, Del Mastro, S, Fraschini, F (1979) Attuali orientamenti della chemioterapia nelle infezioni da batteri anaerobi. Biol Med 1: 73–88

17. Braga, PC, Del Mastro, S, Fraschini, F (1980) Il metronidazolo nella terapia delle infezioni da batteri anaerobi. Biol Med 2: 207–243

18. Burbige, EJ and Milligan, FD (1975) Pseumembranous colitis. Association with antibiotics and therapy with cholestyramine. J Am Med Assoc 231: 1157–1158

19. Cameron, A, Thomas, M (1977) Pseudomembranous colitis and co-trimoxazole. Br Med J 1: 1321–1323

20. Chang, TW, Onderdonk, AB, Bartlett, JG (1978) Anion exchange resins in antibiotic-associated colitis. Lancet 2: 258–259

21. Chang, TW, Garbadi, SL, Bartlett, JG, Saginur, R (1990) Bacitracin treatment of antibiotic-associated colitis and diarrhea caused by Clostridium difficile toxin. Gastroenterology 78: 1584–1586

22. Cohen, MH (1976) Effect of oral prophylactic broad spectrum nonadsorbable antibiotics on the gastrointestinal absorption of nutrients and methotrexate in small cell bronchogenic carcinoma patients. Cancer 38: 1556–1601

23. Cudmore, M, Silva, J, Fekety, R (1980) Clostridial enterocolitis produced by antineoplastic agents in hamsters and humans. Curr Chemother Infect Dis 2: 1460–1463

24. Drasar, BS, Barrow, PA (1985) Intestinal microbiology. American Society for Microbiology, Washington

25. Dukes, MMG (ed) (1988) Meyler's side effects of drugs. Elsevier, Amsterdam

26. Edlund, C, Nord, CE (1986) Comparative in vitro activities of ciprofloxacin enoxacin, norfloxacin, ofloxacin and pefloxacin against Bacteroides fragilis and Clostridium difficile. Scand J Infect Dis 18: 149–151

27. Fee, HJ, Ament, ME, Holmes, EC (1977) Pseudomembranous colitis associated with cephazolin therapy. Am J Surg 133: 247–251

28. Fekety, R, O'Connor, R, Silva, J (1983) Rifampin and pseudomembranous colitis. Rev Infect Dis 5 (Suppl 3) 524

29. Finegold, SM (1970) Interaction of antimicrobial therapy and intestinal flora. Am J Clin Nutr 23: 1466–1471

30. Finegold, SM, Posnick, DJ, Miller, KLG, Hewitt, WL (1965) The effects of various antibacterial compounds on the normal human fecal flora. Ernährungsforschung 10: 316–341

31. Finegold, SM, Davis, A, Miller, LG (1967) Comparative effect of broad-spectrum antibiotics on nonspore-forming anaerobes and normal bowel flora. Ann New York Acad Sci 145: 268–281

32. Friedman, GD, Gerard, MJ, Ury, HK (1976) Clindamycin and diarrhoea. J Am Med Assoc 236: 2498–2501

33. George, WL, Rolfe, RD, Harding, GKM et al. (1982) Clostridium difficile from the environment and contacts of patients with antibiotic-associated colitis. J Infect Dis 143: 40–48

34. Grünenberg, RN, Ridgway, GL, Cremer, AWF, Felmingham, D (1983) The sensitivity of gram-positive pathogens to teichomycin and vancomycin. Drug Exp Clin Res 9: 139–141

35. Heimdahl, A, Nord, CE (1983) Influence of doxycycline on the normal human flora and colonization of the oral cavity and colon. Scand J Infect Dis 15: 293–302
36. Heimdahl, A, Nord, CE (1979) Effect of phenoxymethylpenicillin and clindamycin on the oral, throat an fecal microflora of man. Scand J Infect Dis 11: 233–242
37. Heimdahl, A, Nord, CE (1982) Effect of erythromycin and clindamycin on the indigenous human anaerobic flora and new colonisation of the intestinal tract. Eur J Clin Micr 1: 38–48
38. Kager, L, Ljungdahl, I, Malmborg, AS, Nord, CE (1981) Effect of imidazole prophylaxis on the normal macroflora in patients undergoing colorectal surgery. Scand J of Infect Dis 26: 84–91
39. Kager, L, Malmborg, AS, Sjostedt, S, Nord, CE (1983) Concentrations of ampicillin plus sulbactam in serum and intestinal mucosa and on the colonic microflora in patients undergoing colorectal surgery. Eur J Clin Micr 2: 559–563
40. Kager, L, Malmborg, AS, Nord, CE (1983) Impact of short-term as compared with long-term prophylaxis with cefoxitin on the colonic microflora in patients undergoing colorectal surgery. Drugs Exptl Clin Res 9: 387–392
41. Kager, L, Malmborg, AS, Nord, CE, Sjostedt, S (1983) The effect of piperacillin prophylaxis on the colonic microflora in patients undergoing colorectal surgery. Infection 11: 251–254
42. Kager, L, Brismar, B, Malmborg, AS, Nord, CE (1985) Effect of aztreonam on the colon microflora in patients undergoing colorectal surgery. Infection 13: 111–114
43. Keighley, MRB, Burdon, DW, Arabi, Y et al. (1978) Randomised trial of vancomycin for pseudomembranous colitis and post-operative diarrhea. Brit Med J 2: 1667–1669
44. Keighley, MRB, Burdon, DW, Alexander-Williams, J et al. (1978) Diarrhoea and pseudomembranous colitis after gastrointestinal operations. Lancet 2, 1165
45. Knothe, H (1963) Darmflora und Antibiotika unter besonderer Berücksichtigung der Tetracycline. Deutscher Medizinische Wochenschrift 88: 1469–1477
46. Knothe, H, Wiedermann, B (1965) Die Wirkung von Ampicillin auf die Darmflora des gesunden Menschen. Zentralblatt Bakteriologie 1 Abt Orig 197: 234–243
47. Kuceys, A, Bennet, N, MCK (1989) The use of antibiotics. Heineman Medical Books, Oxford, pp 1064–1072
48. Leigh, DA, Simmons, K (1978) Effect of clindamycin and lincomycin therapy of faecal flora. J Clin Pathol 31: 439–443
49. Lindenbaum, J, Rund, DG, Butler, VP, Jr et al. (1981) Inactivation of digoxin by the gut flora, reversal by antibiotic therapy. N Engl J Med 305: 789–794
50. Lombardi, P, Goldin, B, Bontin, E, Gorbach, SL (1978) Metabolism of androgens and estrogens by human fecal microorganisms. J Steroid Biochem 9: 795–801
51. Matuchousky, C, Aries, J, Maire, P (1978) Metromidazole for antibiotic associated pseudomembranous colitis. Lancet 2: 580–581
52. Mogg, GM, Keighley, M, Burdon, D, et al. (1979) Antibiotic-associated colitis, a review of 66 cases. Br J Surg 66: 738–742
53. Newsom, SWB, Matthews, J, Rampling, AM (1985) Susceptibility of clostridium difficile strains to new antibiotics: quinolones, efrotomycin, teicoplanin and imipenem. J Antimicr Chemother 15: 648–649
54. Noble, JT, Barza, M (1985) Pharmacokinetic properties of the newer cephalosporins. A valid basis for drug selection? Drugs 30: 175–181
55. Nord, CE, Heimdahl, A, Kager, I, Malmborg, AS (1984) The impact of different antimicrobial agents on the normal gastrointestinal flora. Rev Infec Dis 6 (Suppl 1): S 270–S 275
56. Nord, CE, Kager, L, Philipsson, A, Stiernstedt, G (1984) Impact of imipenem/cilastatin therapy on faecal flora. Eur J Clin Microbiol 3: 475–477

57. Nord, CE, Bergan, T, Aase, S (1986) Impact of azlocillin on the colon micro-flora. Scand J Infect Dis 18: 163–166
58. Nord, CE, Heimdahl, A, Kager, L (1986) Antimicrobial induced alterations of the human oropharyngeal and intestinal microflora. Scand J Infect Dis 49 (Suppl): 64–72
59. Oldenbuirger, TR, Miller, MS (1980) Treatment of pseudomembranous colitis with oral metroidazole after relapse following vancomycin. Am J Gastroenterol 74: 359–360
60. Pantosti, A, Luzzi, I, Cardines, R, Gianfrilli, P (1985) Comparison of the in vitro activities of teicoplanin and vancomycin against Clostridium difficile and their interactions with cholestyramine. Antimicr Angets Chemother 28: 847–848
61. Pashby, NL, Bolton, RP, Sherriff, RJ (1979) Oral metronidazole in Clostridium difficile colitis. Br Med J 1: 1605–1606
62. Read, L, Cave-Smith, JR (1977) Pseudomembranous enterocolitis complicating ampicillin therapy. Postgrad Med J 53: 324–327
63. Reeves, DS (1986) The effect of quinolone antibacterials on the gastrointestinal flora compared with that of other antibacterials. J Antimicr Chemoth 18 (Suppl D): 89–102
64. Reimers, D, Nopcke-Fink, L, Brever, H (1974) Rifampin and "pill" do not go well together. J Am Med Ass 227: 608
65. Ripa, S, Mignini, F, Prenna, M, Falcioni, E (1987) In vitro antibacterial activity of rifaximin against Clostridium difficile, Compylobacter jejunii and Yersinia spp. Drugs Exp Clin Res 13: 483–488
66. Robertson, MB, Breen, KJ, Desmond, PV et al. (1977) Incidence of antibiotic-related diarrhoea and pseudomembranous colitis. Med J Anst 1: 243–247
67. Sagimur, R, Hawley, CR, Bartlett, JG (1980) Colitis associated with metronidazole therapy. J Infect Dis 141: 772–775
68. Sanders, Jr, WE, Sanders, CC (1984) Modification of normal flora by antibiotics: effects on individuals and the environment. In: Root, RK, Saude, MA (eds) New dimensions in antimicrobial therapy. Churchill Livingstone, New York, pp 217–241
69. Sakata, H, Fujita, K, Yoshioka, H (1986) The effect of antimicrobial agents on fecal flora of children. Antimicr Ag Chemother 29: 225–229
70. Savage, DC (1977) Microbial ecology of the gastro-intestinal tract. Ann Rev Microbiol 31: 107–118
71. Savage, DC (1983) Microbial ecology of the gastrointestinal tract. In: Hallgren B (ed) Nutrition and the intestinal flora. Almqvist and Wiksell, Uppsala, pp 17–23
72. Similä, S, Kouvalainen, K, Mäkelä, P (1976) Pseudomembranous colitis after amoxycillin. Lancet 2: 317
73. Sjövall, J, Huitfeldt, B, Magni, L, Nord, CE (1986) Effect of beta-lactam pro-drugs on human intestinal microflora. Scand J Infect Dis 49 (Suppl): 73–83
74. Stanley, RJ, Nelson, GL, Tedesco, FJ (1974) The spectrum of radiographic findings in antibiotic-related pseudo-membranous colitis. Radiology 111: 519–524
75. Stephen, J, Osborne, MP (1988) Pathophysiological mechanisms in diarrhocal disease. In: W Donadie, E Griffiths, J Stephen (eds) Bacteria infections of respiratory and gastrointestinal mucosae. IRL Press for Society for General Microbiology, pp 149–170
76. Tedesco, FJ (1977) Clindamycin and colitis: a review. J Infect Dis 135 (suppl): 95–102
77. Tedesco, FJ (1980) Antibiotic associated PMC. Gastroenterology 78: 192
78. Tedesco, FJ, Stanley, RJ, Alfers, DH (1974) Diagnostic features of clindamycin-associated pseudomembranous colitis. N Engl J Med 290: 841–846
79. Tedesco, FJ, Barton, RW, Alphers, HD (1974) Clyndamycin-associated colitis. Ann Intern Med 81: 429–433
80. Tedesco, FJ, Markham, R, Gurwith, M et al. (1978) Oral vancomycin for antibiotic-associated pseudomembranous colitis. Lancet 2: 226

81. Thomson, G, Clark, AH, Hare, K, Spilg WGS (1981) Pseumembranous colitis after treatment with metronidazole. Br Med J 282: 864–865
82. Tures, JF, Townsend, WF, Rose, HD (1976) Cephalosporin-associated pseudo-membranous colitis. J Am Med Assoc 236: 948–953
83. Van Saene, JJM, Van Saene, HKF, Geitz, JN, Tarko-Smit, NJP, Lerk, CF (1986) Quinolones and colonisation resistance in human volunteers. Pharmaceutish Weekblad Scientific Edition 8: 67–71
84. Wade, JC, de Jough, CA, Newman, KA, Crowley, J, Wiernik, PH, Schimpff, SC (1983) Selective antimicrobial modulation as prophylaxis against infection during granulocytopaenia: trimethoprim-sulfamethoxazole vs nalidixic acid. J Infect Dis 147: 624–634
85. Weinstein, AJ, Alanis, A (1985) Antibiotic side effects. In: Ristuccia AM, Cunha BA (eds) Antimicrobial therapy. Raven, New York
86. Wu, H (1982) Spontaneous persistent pseudomembranous colitis related to Clostridium difficile in ischaemic bowel disease. Br Med J 284: 1606–1610
87. Zintel, HA (1947) Streptomycin in peritonitis. Am J Med 5: 443–448

Laxative-Induced Damage to the Colon

S. MÜLLER-LISSNER

Medizinische Klinik, Klinikum Innenstadt,
Ludwig-Maximilians-Universität München

1 Introduction

Laxatives are among the drugs widely used without prescription. Warnings of their side effects are frequent. Such warnings, however, can hardly be supported by data as long as medication with recommended doses is concerned. This chapter reviews the literature on laxative damage to the colon. However, other side effects are also mentioned.

2 Definition and Classification

No definition of the term laxative is completely satisfactory. If any substance increasing stool volume is called a laxative, natural dietary fiber is also included. If only compounds are meant which act on the absorptive and/or secretory processes of the colonocytes or directly stimulate motility, all osmotic laxatives are excluded. A tentative classification of laxatives with their primary mode of action is presented in Table 1.

Table 1. Classification of laxatives and their mechanism of action

Type	Example	Mode of action
Dietary fiber		
Digestible (microflora)	Pectin	Increased bacterial mass
Not digestible	Bran	Water binding
Unabsorbable sugars and sugar alcohols	Lactulose, lactitol, mannitol	Osmotic water binding by compound and split products
Salinic laxatives	$MgSO_4$, MgOH	Osmotic water binding
Anthraquinones	Sennoside A, B	Antiabsorptive/secretagogue and prokinetic on colon
Diphenyl methane derivatives	Bisacodyl, Na-picosulfate	Antiabsorptive/secretagogue and prokinetic on colon
Fatty acids[a]	Rhicinoleic acid	Antiabsorptive/secretagogue and prokinetic on small and large intestine
Dihydroxy bile acids[a]	Deoxycholic acid	Antiabsorptive/secretagogue on colon
5-HT$_4$ antagonists	Cisapride	Prokinetic on colon

[a] Should not be used for chronic constipation.

The in vivo situation is more complex since changes of absorption/secretion induce changes in colonic motility and vice versa. Most work has been done on anthraquinones and diphenyl methane derivatives. Their structural formulas are shown in Fig. 1 and 2. These are also the drugs most frequently involved in laxative abuse.

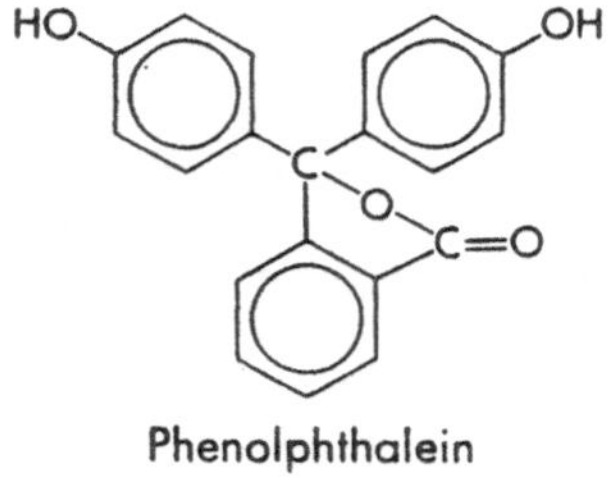

Phenolphthalein

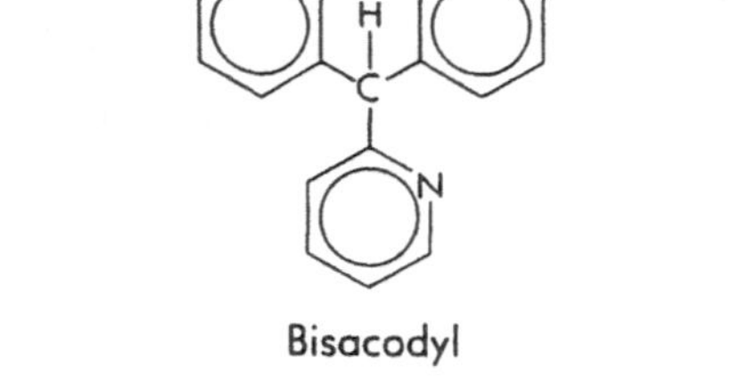

Bisacodyl

Fig. 1. Structure of the diphenyl methane derivatives (diphenolic laxatives). Sodium picosulfate has sodium sulfate groups instead of acetyl groups

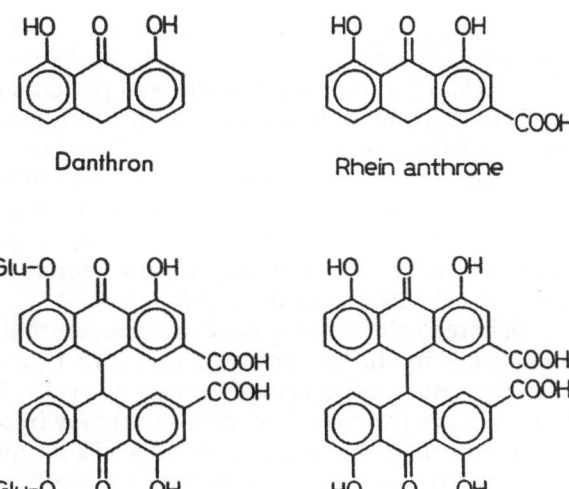

Fig. 2. Structures of the anthraquinones. Binding of two anthraquinone molecules leads to one sennidine molecule. There are symmetric (sennidines A and B) and asymmetric forms (sennidines C and D). Natural forms of the sennidines are glycosilated (sennosides). These are split by colonic bacteria to aglycones and then to the active component rhein anthrone

3 Laxative-Induced Injury to the Colon

3.1 Damage to Surface Epithelium

In constipated patients with chronic intake of various laxatives, a rarefication and change in shape of the microvilli, damage to mitochondria, and increase in the number of lysosomes of colonocytes has been found [3, 41]. These changes were not observed in a group of untreated controls [41]. Furthermore, plication of the lateral cell membrane with widening of the intracellular space and granular inclusions within the colonocytes has been observed [3, 15]. Experimentally, laxation by either bisacodyl or phosphate enemas induces damage to the villi, disappearance of goblet cells, and superficial erosions in healthy volunteers [31]. The same holds true for rhein, bisacodyl, and phenolphthalein in the guinea pig colon [51]. In guinea pigs, danthrone leads to apoptosis of colonocytes: chromatin is seen at the periphery of the cell, and the cells migrate in the intercryptal region [55]. (In contrast, in the process of normal cell turnover, cells are shed mostly into the colonic lumen.)

3.2 Melanosis Coli

This consists of a darkbrown discoloration of the colonic mucosa which begins abruptly at the ileocolonic junction and may extend to the dentate line. The intensity is highest in the cecum and fades in the aboral direction [28]. It may increase again in the rectum [16]: The prevalence of the macroscopically visible melanosis in proctoscopic series is between 1% and 8% [3, 5, 16]. Melanosis has been observed in 12%–31% of unselected constipated patients [2, 5].

The morphological basis of melanosis is pigment within macrophages of the colonic mucosa [56]. The underlying pigment is probably lipofuscin, but it has not exactly been characterized [35, 54]. Therefore, the terms pseudomelanosis and pseudofuscinosis have been proposed instead of melanosis and lipofuscinosis, respectively. However, these terms are no more accurate and are clumsier. Hence, the usual term "melanosis" may be maintained.

Whereas the macrophages of the normal colon are found almost exclusively in the submucosa, they are located above the muscularis mucosae and between crypts in melanosis [3, 52]. Such pigment-loaded macrophages (microscopic melanosis) may be seen up to ten times more frequently than the macroscopically visible melanosis [2, 3, 56]. In an autopsy series, microscopic melanosis was found in 60% of cases [28]. Microscopic melanosis has also been described in the terminal ileum [56]. Probably the same pigment but in larger granules has also been found in macrophages within mesenteric lymph nodes in patients with melanosis coli [17, 56].

A correlation between the intake of laxatives, in particular that of anthraquinones, and melanosis was first described in 1933 by Bockus et al., and the correlation is generally accepted now [2, 3, 16, 50]. A causal relation between intake of anthraquinones and melanosis has also been confirmed experimentally in man and experimental animals. In a case-control study, constipated patients were treated with sennosides or salinic laxatives in alternating time periods, and the development and disappearance of melanosis was followed [50]. Sennosides produced melanosis within 4–13 months in each patient, which disappeared within 5–11 months after switching to the salinic laxative. Furthermore, administration of sennosides or danthrone to guinea pigs does not only lead to apoptosis, but in addition pigmented macrophages can be found between crypts as well as above and below the muscularis mucosae. In these macrophages, pyknotic cell debris may be observed [45, 51, 55]. With a certain delay, the macrophages are seen in the mesenteric lymph nodes [55]. Pigmented macrophages are also found following a 10-day treatment of guinea pigs with bisacodyl or phenolphthalein (Spiessens et al. 1991). A microscopic melanosis is found in 52% of patients with anthraquinone intake and in 8% of those with intake of other laxatives [2]. A clearcut relation between the duration of intake or dose of the laxative and the degree of melanosis could not be established.

The above findings may be summarized as follows (Fig. 3). The mentioned laxatives damage the colonocytes, which migrate into the intercryptal space (apoptosis). After phagocytosis by macrophages, a lipofuscinlike pigment is generated, which stains the mucosa dark brown if occurring in larger amounts. If cell damage subsides, melanosis de-

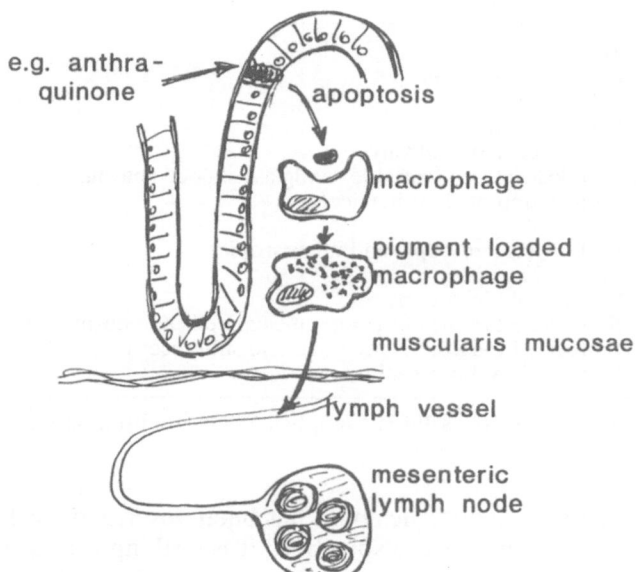

e.g. anthra-
quinone

apoptosis

macrophage

pigment loaded
macrophage

muscularis mucosae

lymph vessel

Fig.3. Schematic
representation of
the pathogenesis of
melanosis coli

mesenteric
lymph node

creases slowly since the macrophages migrate toward the mesenteric lymph nodes. This process is particularly pronounced during intake of anthraquinones but also occurs during intake of at least bisacodyl and phenolphthalein. There is no indication that melanosis has any pathophysiologic consequences.

3.3 Cathartic Colon

This is an abnormality of the colon which has been defined on the basis of radiologic findings in patients with chronic laxative intake. Morphologically, changes of both mucosa and submucosa are found (Table 2). It was first described in 1943 by Heilbrun. A total of 27 cases have been reported which fulfill the criteria listed in Table 2 [1, 9, 10, 19, 20, 23, 25, 30, 36, 53]. One third of these were described by Heilbrun and Bernstein [20]; three other publications describe eight further cases of "cathartic colon" which do not fulfill the mentioned criteria [14, 37, 46].

Upon analysis of the 27 cases it becomes apparent that exclusively women were affected who had taken laxatives for chronic constipation over 1–7 decades. The doses used were in the therapeutic range. All patients mentioned the laxative intake spontaneously. Further, at least one decade of laxative intake fell in the 50s or earlier. No case has been published in which laxative intake began after 1960. Finally, among published cases of laxative abuse using high doses of laxatives, which have been reported almost exclusively during the past 3 decades, not a single

Table 2. Morphologic characteristics of the cathartic colon

Barium enema
   Loss of haustration
   Dilated lumen
   Dilated terminal ileum
   Gaping of ileocecal valve
   Pseudostrictures (variable sandglass-shaped spasms)
   Predilection of right hemicolon

Pathology (macroscopic and microscopic)
   Mucosal atrophy
   Superficial ulcerations
   Submucosal infiltrates (mononuclear cells and eosinophils)
   Fibrosis of muscularis mucosae and submucosa
   Increase in submucosal fat

(After Avery Jones 1967; Campbell 1983; Heilbrun and Bernstein 1955; Kim et al. 1978; Urso et al. 1975)

case of true cathartic colon has been described. In 19 of the 27 cases the laxatives taken were specified; it is striking that at least 17 of the 19 patients had taken podophyllin. Besides podophyllin, aloe and cascara preparations, in one case kalomel and a number of plant extracts were taken. Podophyllin is a poison of the metaphase of the cell cycle which induces ulcerations and neuropathies when applied topically [7]. Acute intake of large amounts may induce a sensomotor neuropathy and a psychosyndrome [11].

Therefore the conclusion seems attractive that the cathartic colon may have been induced by laxative compounds, principally by podophyllin, which are now no longer used.

3.4 Damage to the Autonomous Nervous System

With respect to this topic, conflicting results have been obtained, both in laboratory animals and in constipated patients. The probably most frequently cited experimental study was performed in mice with oral and intraperitoneal administration of a senna sirup [48]. Unfortunately, details of the methodology (composition of the sirup, dose, duration of treatment) as well as data are lacking. A time-dependent "degeneration" of nerve fibers is reported after silver staining. In contrast, no changes were found in mice treated daily with 10 mg/kg sennosides orally for 4 months using the electron microscope [12]. Negative results were also obtained in rats after a 6-month treatment with 25 or 100 mg/kg sennosides daily [44]. With a similar experimental procedure no damage to the colonic nerve plexuses or immunohistochemical changes were found in rats or mice. However, in mice there was an unexpected increase in the count of neurons, the meaning of which is unclear [24].

It has been speculated that the senna sirup mentioned above might have contained free (i.e., not glycosilated) anthraquinones. These are absorbed in the small intestine and might be systemically toxic. Therefore, rats were treated with a high dose (250 mg/kg daily) of danthrone (1,8-dihydroxy anthraquinone) for 4 months. In all treated animals, but not in controls, axonal damage was found, which was severe in 40 % of cases [12]. These findings were not reproduced with a lower dose (80 mg/kg daily for 4 months) [21]. Pretreatment with a low dose of danthrone, and possibly also with sennosides, induced changes in mesenteric vascular resistance, the meaning of which also remains unclear [38].

An increased diameter of axons and a reduction in neurofilaments was found in constipated patients who took a variety of laxatives for years, in comparison to patients with the irritable bowel syndrome and in comparison to healthy controls [42]. Furthermore, swollen axons with electron-dense inclusions were found in such patients [3] as well as lysosomes within neurons and Schwann's cells [52]. Also using silver staining, abnormalities of the nerve plexus of constipated patients have been described [29, 49]. Finally, in patients with slow colonic transit a reduced or totally lacking reaction of the enteric nerves with a neurofilament-specific antibody has been observed [27]. Only one study compares the morphology of the autonomous nervous system of constipated patients taking anthraquinones (aloe) to that of an appropriate control group of constipated patients without laxative intake. These authors found no relevant differences with respect to the electron microscopic appearance [40].

In summary, the arguments in favor of laxative-induced damage to the autonomous nervous system of the colon have been obtained on the basis of poorly documented experiments and are restricted to silver staining of nerve fibers. Studies which show damage to be unlikely are well documented and use a variety of techniques, but not silver stains. Morphological damage to the autonomous nerve system of the colon by sennosides in glycosidic binding and clinically relevant dose has been shown neither in experimental animals nor in man. The studies in patients do not allow a final conclusion as to whether the abnormalities observed are a consequence of laxative intake, or whether they represent preexisting changes of unknown etiology which lead to slow colonic transit which in turn leads the patient to take laxative.

3.5 Functional Impairment

Any relevant damage to the autonomous nervous system should result in an impairment of function. Therefore it is of interest whether any findings suggest disordered absorption or motility of the colon induced by laxatives.

Chronic treatment with sennosides has no effect on spontaneous contractile activity of the rat colon in vitro [34]. Bisacodyl in doses which induce diarrhea increases the serum aldosterone levels [4]. Since aldosterone increases sodium absorption, bisacodyl is less effective on water and sodium secretion after chronic pretreatment than without such pretreatment [4]. Accordingly, the efficacy of rhein, bisacodyl, and phenolphthalein decreases during 10-day treatment in guinea pigs [51].

The development of tolerance to laxatives has not properly been studied in patients. However, a couple of studies do not show a loss of effect of laxatives. Instead, a proportion of the patients with chronic laxative intake could be switched to dietary fiber [13, 18, 26], rectal laxatives [57], or cisapride [32] without further need for oral laxatives. However, there are occasional patients with documented slow-transit constipation who report a need to increase the dose of laxative in order to maintain the desired effect.

4 Other Untoward Effects of Laxatives when Taken in Recommended Doses

4.1 Abdominal Complaints

These may occur with all types of laxatives. Since constipation by itself is often associated with abdominal complaints, the causative role of the laxative is not always apparent. Compounds which can be digested by the colonic microflora produce mainly meteorism and flatulence. Sennosides and diphenylmethane derivatives may lead to cramping abdominal pain. In a controlled study this was three times more frequent than with placebo treatment [47].

4.2 Changes in Serum Electrolytes

In prospective studies over more than 1 year in 139 patients, no changes in serum electrolyte levels, in particular potassium, were found with recommended doses of sennosides [22, 43]. When salinic laxatives are used, however, substantial amounts of electrolytes may be absorbed. This is particularly relevant in patients with impaired renal function in whom hypermagnesemia has been observed [26].

5 Laxative Abuse

Besides diuretics, laxatives are among the drugs with a relatively high rate of abuse, particularly in patients with anorexia nervosa, bulimia, and Münchhausen's syndrome. The frequency of laxative-induced diarrhea among 200 patients with diarrhea was 3.5 % [8]. In another study in 27 patients with diarrhea in whom a diagnostic procedure did not reveal a cause, laxative intake was eventually uncovered in 25 % [39].

The literature on case reports of hidden laxative use comprises approximately 70 publications with 150 cases [33]. With few exceptions, patients were hospitalized for diarrhea of unknown origin, weight loss, abdominal pain, or muscular weakness (due to hypokalemia). Laxative intake was usually admitted only after confrontation with a positive finding at a locker search or with a positive assay in urine. The reported doses are therefore to be interpreted with caution. They are scattered over a wide range of up to 200 doses per day. The preferred drugs are phenolphthalein, plant extracts containing anthraquinones, and bisacodyl. More than 95 % of the patients were female. The following side effects have been observed in such patients but not in prospective studies with recommended doses of laxatives.

Hypokalemia is the most common finding. This is explained by fecal loss that is aggravated by secondary hyperaldosteronism, which is in turn due to losses of water and sodium. As long as kidney function is not impaired, hypokalemia leads to metabolic alkalosis (Fig. 4). Potassium depletion reduces the concentration ability of the renal tubules and lowers the clearances of inulin, creatinin, and *para*-aminohippurie acid. Histologically, the epithelium of the tubules exhibits degenerative changes which are at least partially reversible.

A frequent reason for laxative abuse is attempted weight loss. Although short-term laxative intake may reduce body weight by loss of water, it is not apparent why and how chronic intake should be effective.

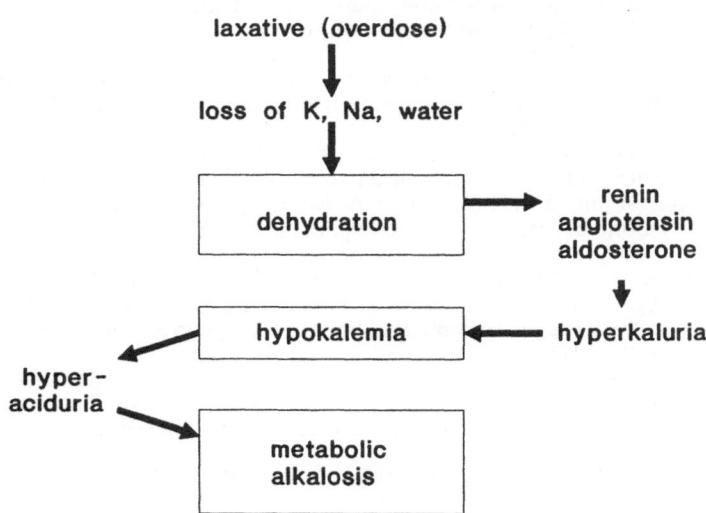

Fig. 4. Metabolic consequences of laxative abuse

However, a slight malabsorption of nutrients has been documented in volunteer studies, but the underlying mechanisms have not been elucidated [6].

In some case reports, finger clubbing in association with abuse of anthraquinones has been described.

6 Conclusion

Well-documented morphologic changes of the colon due to laxatives are melanosis coli and the cathartic colon. Melanosis coli is due to pigment-loaded macrophages within the submucosa. It occurs mainly after long-term intake of anthraquinone-containing preparation. The cathartic colon is characterized by dilatation, loss of haustration, and pseudostrictures. It apparently has not been observed in recent decades; therefore it was probably caused by laxatives that are no longer used. Current evidence is more against than in favor of damage to the autonomous nervous system of the colon by the laxatives currently used.

Acknowledgement. This research was supported by Deutsche Forschungsgemeinschaft, Grant Mu 629/2-3.

References

1. Avery Jones, F (1967) Cathartic colon. Proc R Soc Med 60: 503–550
2. Badiali, MD, Marcheggiano, A, Pallone, F, Paoluzi, P, Bausano G, Iannoni, C, Materia, E, Anzini, F, Corazziari, E (1985) Melanosis of the rectum in patients with chronic constipation. Dis Colon Rectum 28: 241–245
3. Balász, M (1986) Melanosis coli. Ultrastructural study of 45 patients. Dis Colon Rectum 29: 839–844
4. Beubler, E (1985) Influence of chronic bisacodyl treatment on the effect of acute bisacodyl on water and electrolyte transport in the rat colon. J Pharm Pharmacol 37: 131–133
5. Bockus, HL, Williard, JH, Bank, J (1933) Melanosis coli. The etiologic significance of the anthracene laxatives. A report of forty-one cases. JAMA 101: 1–6
6. Bo-Linn, GW, Santa Ana, CA, Morawsky, SW, Fordtran; JS (1983) Purging and calorie absorption in bulimic patients and normal women. Ann Intern Med 99: 14–17
7. Brunton, LL (1990) Agents affecting gastrointestinal water flux and motility, digestants, and bile acids. In: Goodman Gilman, A, Rall, TW, Nies, AS, Taylor, P (eds) The pharmacological basis of therapeutics, 8th edn. Pergamon, New York pp 914–932
8. Bytzer, P, Stokholm, M, Andersen, I, Klitgaard, NA, Schaffalitzky, DE, Muckadell, OB (1989) Prevalence of surreptitious laxative abuse in patients with diarrhoea of uncertain origin: a cost benefit analysis of a screening procedure. Gut 30: 1379–1384
9. Campbell, WL (1983) Cathartic colon. Reversibility of roentgen changes. Dis Colon Rectum 26: 445–448
10. Diller, WF (1965) Röntgenologische Aspekte des "Abführmittelcolons." Dtsch Med Wochenschr 90: 478–483

11. Dobb, GJ, Edis, RH (1984) Coma and neuropathy after ingestion of herbal laxative containing podophyllin. Med J Aust 140: 495–496
12. Dufour, P, Gendre, P. (1984) Ultrastructure of mouse intestinal mucosa and changes observed after long-term anthraquinone administration. Gut 15: 1358–1363
13. Franken, FH, Wiechers, B (1975) Melanosis coli. Leber Magen Darm 5, 269–271
14. Geboes, K, Bossaert, H (1980) Cathartic colon – two case reports. Am J Proctol 31: 21–24
15. Ghadially, FN, Parry, EW (1966) An electron-microscope and histochemical study of melanosis coli. J Path Bact 92: 313–317
16. Göbel, D (1978) Melanosis coli. Med Klin 73: 519–523
17. Hall, M, Eusebi, V (1978) Yellow-brown spindle bodies in mesenteric lymph nodes: a possible relationship with melanosis coli. Histopathology 2: 47–52
18. Haward, LRC, Hughes-Roberts, HE (1962) The treatment of constipation in mental hospitals. Gut 3: 85–90
19. Heilbrun, N (1943) Roentgen evidence suggesting enterocolitis associated with prolonged cathartic abuse. Radiology 41: 486–491
20. Heilbrun, N, Bernstein, C (1955) Roentgen abnormalities of the large and small intestine associated with prolonged carthagic ingestion. Radiology 65: 549–556
21. Heinicke, EA, Kiernan, JA (1990) Resistance of myenteric neurons in the rat colon to depletion by 1,8-dihydroxyanthraquinone. J Pharm Pharmacol 42: 123–125
22. Heiny, BM (1976) Langzeitbehandlung mit einem pflanzlichen Laxativum. Serumelektrolyte und Säurenbasenhaushalt. Ärztliche Praxis 28: 563–564
23. Jewell, FC, Kline, JR (1954) The purged colon. Radiology 62: 368–370
24. Kiernan, JA, Heinicke, EH (1989) Sennosides do not kill myenteric neurons in the colon of the rat or mouse. Neuroscience 30: 837–842
25. Kim, SK, Gerle, RD, Rozanski, R (1978) Cathargic colitis. Am J Roentgenol 131: 1079–1081
26. Kinnunen, O, Salokannel, J (1987) Constipation in elderly long-stay patients: its treatment by magnesium hydroxyde and bulk laxative. Ann Clin Res 19: 321–323
27. Klück, P, ten Kate, FJW, Schouten, WR, Bartels, KCM, Tibboel, D, van der Kamp, AWM, Molenaar, JC, van Blankenstein, M (1987) Efficacy of antibody NF2F11 staining in the investigation of severe long-standing constipation. Gastroenterology 93: 872–875
28. Koskela, E, Kulju, T, Collan, Y (1989) Prevalence, distribution, and histologic features in 200 consecutive autopsies at Kuopio University Central Hospital. Dis Colon Rectum 32: 235–239
29. Krishnamurthy, S, Schuffler, MD, Rohrmann, CA, Pope, CE (1985) Severe idiopathic constipation is associated with a distinctive abnormality of the colonic myenteric plexus. Gastroenterol 88: 26–34
30. Lemaitre, G, L'Herminé, C, Decoulx, M, Houcke, M, Linquette, M (1970) Aspect radiologique des colites chroniques par abus de laxatifs à propos de quatre observations. J Belge Radiologie 53: 339–345
31. Meisel, JL, Bergman, D, Graney, D, Saunders, DR, Rubin, CE (1977) Human rectal mucosa: proctoscopic and morphological changes caused by laxatives. Gastroenterol 72: 1274–1279
32. Müller-Lissner, SA, Bavarian Constipation Study Group (1987) Treatment of chronic constipation with cisapride and placebo. Gut 28: 1033–1038
33. Müller-Lissner, SA (1992) Nebenwirkungen von Laxantien. Z Gastroenterol 30: 418–427
34. Odenthal, KP, Ziegler, D (1988) In vitro effects of anthraquinones on rat intestine and uterus. Pharmacology 36: 57–65
35. Park, C, Cho, NH, Jeong, HJ (1990) Histochemical and immunohistochemical comparison of the pigments of melanosis coli and Dubin-Johnson syndrome. Yonsei Med J 31: 27–32

36. Plum, GE, Weber, HM, Sauer, WG (1960) Prolonged cathartic abuse resulting in roentgen evidence suggestive of enterocolitis. Am J Roentgenol 83: 919–925
37. Plumley, PF (1973) Radical surgery in the treatment of carthatic colon. Proc R Soc Med 66: 243–244
38. Ralevic, V, Hoyle, CHV, Burnstock, G (1990) Effects of long-term laxative treatment on rat mesenteric resistance vessel responses in vitro. Gastroenterol 99: 1352–1357
39. Read, NW, Krejs, GJ, Read, MG (1980) Chronic diarrhea of unknown origin. Gastroenterol 78: 264–271
40. Riecken, EO, Zeitz, M, Emde, C, Hopert, R, Witzel, L, Hintze, R, Marsch-Ziegler, U, Vester, JC (1990) The effect of an anthraquinone laxative on colonic nerve tissue: a controlled trial in constipated women. Z Gastroenterol 28: 660–664
41. Riemann, JF, Schenk, J, Ehler, R, Schmidt, H, Koch, H (1978) Ultrastructural changes of colonic mucosa in patients with chronic laxative misuse. Acta Hepato-Gastroenterol 25: 213–218
42. Riemann, JF, Schmidt, H, Zimmermann, W (1980) The fine structure of colonic submucosal nerves in patients with chronic laxative abuse. Scand J Gastroent 15: 761–768
43. Rosprich, G, Dauerbehandlung mit Laxantien (1980) Therapiewoche 30: 5836–5837
44. Rudolph, RL, Mengs, U (1988) Electron microscopical studies on rat intestine after long-term treatment with sennosides. Pharmacology 36 (Suppl 1): 188–193
45. Russel, NJ, Royland, JE, McCawley, EL (1980) Danthron induced melanosis coli in guinea pig. Proc West Pharmacol Soc 23: 277–280
46. Schmidt, H, Riemann, JF, Rödl, W (1983) Megakolon nach langährigem Laxantienabusus. Med Klin Prax 78: 62/64/76
47. Shelton, MG (1980) Standardized senna in the management of constipation in the puerperium. S Afr Med J 57: 78–80
48. Smith, B (1969) Effect of irritant purgatives on the myenteric plexus in man and the mouse. Gut 9: 139–143
49. Smith, B (1973) Pathologic changes in the colon produced by anthraquinone purgatives. Dis Colon Rectum 16: 465–468
50. Speare, GS (1951) Melanosi coli. Experimental observations on its production and elimination in twenty-tree cases. Am J Surg 82: 631–637
51. Spiessens, C, De Witte, D, Geboes, K, Lemli, J (1991) Experimental inductium of pseudomelanosis coli by anthromoid laxatives monanthronoid laxatives. Pharmaceut Pharmacol Lett 1: 3–6
52. Steer, HW, Colin-Jones, DG (1975) Melanosis coli: studies of the toxic effects of irritant purgatives. J Path 115: 199–205
53. Urso, FP, Urso, MJ, Lee, CH (1975) The cathartic colon: pathological findings and radiological/pathological correlation. Radiology 116: 557–560
54. Vogel, A, Fabricius, W, Dulce, HJ, Stolpmann, HJ (1969) Zur Struktur und Herkunft des Pigmentes bei der Melanosis coli. Virchows Arch Abt A Path Anat 346: 74–88
55. Walker, NI, Bennet, RE, Axelsen, RA (1988) A consequence of anthraquinone-induced apoptosis of colonic epithelial cells. Amer J Pathology 131: 465–476
56. Wittoesch, JH, Jackman, RJ, McDonald, JR (1958) Melanosis coli: general review and a study of 887 cases. Dis Colon Rectum 1: 172–180
57. Wolcott L (1963) Laxation in patients with chronic disease utilizing bisacodyl. Arch Phys Med Rehabil 44: 375–377

Drug-Induced Injuries of the Liver and Biliary Tract

D. LARREY

Service d'Hépato-gastroentérologie,
Hôpital Saint-Eloi, Montpellier, France

---

1 Introduction

Hepatic and biliary drug reactions have been increasingly recognized as major causes of liver and biliary tract diseases over the last 20 years [37, 66, 85, 90]. This may be explained by several factors. First, marked improvements have been made in diagnostic methods (viral serologic tests, ultrasonography, tomodensitometry, magnetic resonance imaging), allowing elimination of other causes of disease and ascertainment of potential involvement of drug reactions more accurately. Thus, the hepatotoxicity of some drugs, such as amiodarone or amodiaquin used for more than 25 years, was only recognized a few years ago [36, 70].

Second, the number of drugs that are potentially toxic has increased to about 600 for the liver [8, 85, 90] and more than 50 for the biliary tract [37, 40]. Furthermore, even medicinal plants may be hepatotoxic [45].

2 Liver Injuries

The spectrum of drug-induced liver injuries is so diverse that almost all liver pathologies may be reproduced [66, 85, 90].

2.1 Acute Hepatitis

2.1.1 Mechanisms

For most drugs, the mechanism behind the hepatotoxicity remains unknown. Toxicity is only rarely due to the parent drug itself; rather, it is frequently related to its transformation into unstable, toxic, reactive metabolites by liver enzymes (for instance, paracetamol, halothane, isoniazid). This metabolic activation is mostly caused by liver cytochrome P-450s. Usually, these metabolites (free radicals or electrophil metabolites) are produced in small amounts and are easily detoxified by various protective mechanisms, in particualar conjugation to glutathione, epoxide hydrolases, glutathione peroxidase, superoxide dismutase, catalase, and suicide inactivation of cytochrome P-450s. When these mechanisms are overwhelmed, reactive metabolites may bind covalently to some hepatocyte constituents including proteins, unsaturated lipids, and nucleic acids. Covalent binding of reactive metabolites can lead to hepatocyte death by interfering with cell homeostasis or by triggering immunological reactions. Consequently, *toxic* and *immunoallergic hepatitis* can occur [66, 85, 90].

There are two types of toxic hepatitis: (1) hepatitis related to overdose in which hepatitis is predictable and frequently fatal (for instance, paracetamol intoxication) [71]. (2) idiosyncratic toxic hepatitis occurring at therapeutic doses; this type is unpredictable and affects a small proportion of treated subjects (1 % or less) (for instance, isoniazid, ketoconazole). For a given patient, hepatitis may recur with the same delay following reexposure to the offending drug under the same circumstances as in the first episode.

Immunoallergic hepatitis is frequently related to a reaction against neoantigens, resulting from the covalent binding of reactive metabolites to hepatocyte constituents present on the plasma membrane [48]. Sometimes, autoimmune phenomena may occur leading to the formation of serum autoantibodies [25]. Some of these antibodies are nonspecific such as anti-smooth muscle or anti-nuclear antibodies (clometacin, papaverine, methyldopa) [25]. Others appear to be specific for a particular drug: type 6 anti-mitochondrial antibodies (iproniazid) [25], type 2 anti-liver/kidney microsome antibodies (anti-LKM2) raised against P-450 2C9 (tienilic acid, so-called ticrynafen) [5] and anti-liver microsome antibodies (anti-LM) raised against P-450 1A2 (dihydralazine) [10].

Drug hepatotoxicity may be promoted by varying factors [67]: *Starvation and malnutrition* can decrease the amount of hepatic glutathione necessary for detoxification of reactive metabolites (paracetamol, for instance). This might explain the greater frequency of some types of drug-induced hepatitis in patients with AIDS (hepatitis caused by dapsone or by sulfamethoxazole-trimethoprim combination) [27]. *Enzymatic induction* by one drug may increase the transformation rate of another drug into reactive metabolites; for example, rifampicin increases isoniazid toxicity and chronic alcoholism that of paracetamol [77]. As a result of *genetic factors* [67], a low sulfoxidation capacity may increase chlorpromazine hepatotoxicity; a low acetylation capacity increases sulfonamide hepatotoxicity; a deficiency in P-450 2D6, responsible for an impairment of debrisoquin/dextromethorphan oxidation capacity, appears to be a major determinant of perhexiline hepatotoxicity [58]; a deficiency in mephenytoin oxidation capacity (P-450 2C9) may influence the risk of developing Atrium hepatotoxicity [26]; a deficiency in detoxification mechanisms of reactive metabolites seems to promote the hepatotoxicity of halothane [20], phenytoin [81], sulfonamides [78] and amineptine [35]; some HLA phenotypes also may modulate drug hepatotoxicity, e.g. HLA A11 for halothane [19], HLA B8 for nitrofurantoin [84] or clometacin [63].

2.1.2 Clinicopathological Features

Acute hepatitis makes up the major form of drug-induced liver injury. A classification of drug-induced acute hepatitis into three types has been recently proposed by an international consensus meeting, based on serum alanine aminotransferase activity (ALT), serum alkaline phosphatase activity (AP), and the ratio ALT/AP expressed as a multiple of the upper limit of the normal value (N) [7]. Despite the absence of direct correlation with histologic features, this classification has the advantage of allowing one to distinguish between various forms of hepatitis with different courses and prognoses [66, 85, 91].

2.1.2.1 Acute Hepatocellular Hepatitis. This type is characterized by a marked increase in ALT levels (over 2N) without an increase in AP, or by ratio > 5 [7]; acute hepatocellular hepatitis generally does not exhibit a specific pattern [66, 85, 91]. Hepatitis may either be asymptomatic or revealed by nonspecific symptoms such as asthenia, anorexia, vomiting, and abdominal pain associated or not with jaundice. Hepatocyte necrosis and lobular inflammation are the major histologic features. Several hundreds of drugs can induce this type of hepatitis (Table 1). In most

Table 1. Main drugs responsible for hepatocellular necrosis (adapted from [66, 85, 90])

Anesthesia	Cardiovascular diseases
Chloroform	Acebutolol
Methoxyflurane	Amiodarone
Fluroxene	Disopyramide
Trichloroethylene	Dihydralazine
Enflurane	Tienilic acid (ticrynafen)
Halothane	Pyridinol carbamate
	Verapamil
Cancer	Labetalol
Carmustine	Methyldopa
Cytarabine	Hydralazine
Moxisylyte	Papaverine
Hydroxycarbamide	Suloctidil
Mitoxantrone	Phenprocoumon
Procarbazine	
Chlorozotocin	Digestive diseases
Dacarbazine	Calcium carbimide
Indicine N-oxide	Disulfiram
Streptozotocin	Salazosulfapyridine
L-Asparaginase	Cyanamide
VP-16	Cimetidine
Cyproterone	Ranitidine
Cyclophosphamide	Dantron
Floxuridine	
Flutamide	Endocrine, nutritional,
6-Mercaptopurine	and metabolic diseases
Vincristine	Acetohexamide

Table 1

Glybuthiazole
Germander
Propylthiouracil
Chlorpropamide
Carbutamide
Metahexamide
Simvastatin
Fenofibrate
Tolbutamide
Gemfibrozil
Cyclofenil

Infectious and parasitic diseases
Aminosalicylic acid
Clindamycin
Ethionamide
Ketoconazole
Mepacrine
Protionamide
Sulfonamide derivatives
Zidovudine
Amodiaquine
Co-trimoxazole
Hycanthone
Levamisole
Oxacillin
Pyrazinamide
Arsenic derivatives
Cloxacillin
Carbenicillin
Dapsone
Isoniazid
Mebendazole
Nitrofurantoin
Piperazine

Neuropsychiatric diseases
Desipramine
Imipramine
Lergotrile
Mebanazine
Nialamide
Phenacemide
Pheniprazine
Viloxazine

Fluoxetine
Zimelidine
Exifone
Loxapine
Atrium
Amitriptyline
Dothiepin
Levodopa
Metiapine
Nomifensine
Pemoline
Phenoxyproperazine
Tetrahydroaminoacridine
Phenelzine
Trazodone
Amineptine
Carbamazepine
Haloperidol
Mianserin
Fipexide
Phenobarbital
Bromocriptine
Iproniazid
Methylphenidate
Phenytoin
Valproic acid

Rheumatic and musculoskeletal
diseases
Allopurinol
Benorilate
Dantrolene
Salicylates
Aspirin
Benoxaprofen
Glafenine
Baclofen
Phenylbutazone
Clometacin
Paracetamol
Pirprofen
Piroxicam

Skin diseases
Etretinate
Methoxsalen

cases withdrawal of the offending drug is followed by prompt clinical improvement and complete recovery within a few weeks, without requiring any treatment. Sometimes, however, liver failure marked by jaundice, severe coagulation disorders, and hepatic encephalopathy may develop. Hepatitis is described as fulminant when the delay between jaundice and encephalopathy is less than 15 days and as subfulminant when it exceeds 15 days. Both fulminant and subfulminant hepatitis are spontaneously fatal in 90 % of patients. Consequently, emergency liver transplantation is now indicated, particularly for young patients [66]. The main causative drugs are paracetamol, halothane, isoniazid, pyrazinamide, and sulfonamides. In paracetamol overdose, hepatitis may be prevented or limited by the prompt administration of *N*-acetylcysteine (4–8 h after paracetamol ingestion) which increases glutathione synthesis [71]. Insidiously, acute hepatocellular hepatitis also can lead to chronic liver disease.

2.1.2.2 Acute Hepatocellular Cholestasis. Characterized by an increase in serum AP levels of over 2N without an abnormality in ALT levels or R < 2 [7], this type of hepatitis includes two subtypes: *pure cholestasis* and *cholestatic hepatitis.*

In pure cholestasis [37, 91], the full clinical picture is comprised of jaundice, pruritus, pale stools, and dark urine. It may be associated with moderate hepatomegaly and xanthomas. Jaundice and pruritus may be lacking. In this case, the diagnosis relies upon biochemical changes and liver biopsy. In addition to high AP activity, biological changes include conjugated hyperbilirubinemia, hypercholesterolemia, and high serum bile acid levels and γ-glutamyltransferase activity. Histologic lesions consist of brownish granular deposits made up of conjugated and unconjugated bilirubin in the hepatocyte cytoplasm. Canaliculi are variably dilated and contain bile pigment material. Cholestasis frequently predominates in the centrilobular area. Pure cholestasis occurs with a few drugs, mainly oral contraceptives, estrogens, and androgens. The risk of developing cholestasis with oral contraceptives is strongly increased by the concomitant administration of troleandomycin, a macrolide antibiotic able to inhibit P-450 3A4 isoenzyme involved in estrogen elimination [56]. Discontinuation of the causative drugs is followed by the disappearance of jaundice and biochemical changes within a few weeks.

The second subtype, cholestatic hepatitis [37, 91], occurs more frequently than pure cholestasis. In addition to pure cholestasis features, it frequently is associated with abdominal pain, fever, chills, and various hypersensitivity manifestations [44]. The clinical syndrome may mimic acute obstruction of the biliary tract, mostly with phenothiazines, macrolides, amineptine, and carbamazepine. Pathological findings are those of pure cholestasis, associated with a small amount of liver cell necrosis, and inflammatory infiltration by mononuclear cells and, sometimes, eosinophils in portal tracts and in the necrotic area. Many drugs may cause cholestatic hepatitis (Table 2); phenothiazines, macrolide antibiotics, tricyclic antidepressants, and nonsteroidal anti-inflammatory drugs (NSAIDS) are typical examples. In most cases, discontinuation of the causative drug is followed by complete recovery within a few weeks. Uncommonly, however, chronic cholestasis with progressive destruction of small bile ducts may develop [13].

Table 2. Main drugs responsible for mixed or cholestatic hepatitis (adapted from [37, 85, 90])

Immunosuppression
  Azathioprine
  Chromomycin A 3
  Cyclosporin
  Thioguanine
  Aminoglutethimide
  Chlorambucil
  Cisplatin
  Mitomycin
  Amsacrine
  Chlorozotocin
  Cytarabine
  Streptozotocin

Cardiovascular diseases
  Ajmaline
  Captropril
  Disopyramide
  Methyldopa
  Papaverine
  Quinidine
  Verapamil
  Aprindine
  Flecainide
  Mexiletine
  Phenindione
  Procainamide
  Warfarin
  Benziodarone
  Diltiazem
  Enalapril
  Hydralazine
  Nifedipine
  Propafenone
  Ticlopidine

Digestive diseases
  Cimetidine
  Penicillamine
  Ranitidine

Endocrine diseases
  Acetohexamide
  Gibenclamide
  Propylthiouracil
  Tolazamide
  Carbimazole
  Metahexamide
  Tamoxifen
  Tolbutamide
  Carbutamide
  Chlopropamide
  Fenofibrate

Methimazole
Thiouracil

Infectious and parasitic diseases
  Aminosalicylic acid
  Cephalosporins
  Cotrimoxazole
  Hycanthone
  Niclofolan
  Troleandomycin
  Penicillin
  Thiabendazole
  Amoxicillin-clavulanic acid
  Chloramphenicol
  Erythromycin derivatives
  Josamycin
  Nitrofurantoin
  Tryparsamide
  Sulfonamide derivatives
  Cabarsone
  Cloxacillin
  Ethambutol
  Griseofulvin
  Ketoconazole
  Nalidixic acid
  Roxithromycin

Neuropsychiatric diseases
  Amitriptyline
  Chlordiazepoxide
  Diazepam
  Haloperidol
  Isocarboxazid
  Phenytoin
  Thioridazine
  Trifluoperazine
  Bromocriptine
  Chlorpromazine
  Fluphenazine
  Imipramine
  Mianserin
  Prochlorperazine
  Trazodone
  Zimelidine
  Carbamazepine
  Desipramine
  Flurazepam
  Iprindole
  Phenobarbital
  Promazine
  Triazolam

Table 2

Rheumatic and musculoskeletal	Penicillamine
diseases	Piroxicam
Allopurinol	Pyritinol
Colchicine	Tolfenamic acid
Fenbufen	Carprofen
Flurbiprofen	Diflunisal
Ibufenac	Gold salts
Oxyphenbutazone	Indomethacin
Phenylbutazone	Niflumic acid
Proquazone	Phenopyrazone
Sulindac	Propoxyphene
Zoxazolamine	Sudoxicam
Baclofen	Probenecid
Diclofenac	Skin diseases
Glafenine	Isotretinoin
Ibuprofen	
Naproxen	

Cholestatic hepatitis is generally ascribed to immunoallergic mechanisms. The observation of several cases of cross-hepatotoxicity between drugs with related chemical structures further supports this view, for example, between phenothiazine derivatives [28]; between tricyclic antidepressants [43]; between erythromycin and troleandomycin [68]; between sulfonamide derivatives [27].

2.1.2.3 Acute Mixed Hepatitis. This term corresponds to acute hepatitis in which both ALT and AP are increased with R between 2 and 5 [6]. The clinical, biological, and pathological picture combines hepatocellular and cholestatic patterns [66, 85, 90]. Jaundice is frequently present. Progression to fulminant hepatitis is unusual. The drugs responsible for mixed hepatitis are very similar to those responsible for hepatocellular or cholestatic hepatitis (Table 2), mainly, tricyclic antidepressants, NSAIDS, macrolide antibiotics, and β-lactamines. The mechanisms involved in mixed hepatitis appear to be mostly immunoallergic.

2.2 Subacute Hepatitis, Chronic Hepatitis, and Cirrhosis

Some drugs can produce prolonged liver cell necrosis resulting in the developement of subacute or chronic liver diseases, such as occur in viral hepatitis. Prolonged necrosis may occur in four circumstances [66]: (1) The liver lesions may develop silently for several months or may be responsible for only mild and nonspecific symptoms such as asthenia. As a consequence, liver injury is detected and treatment is continued. When the liver disease is eventually recognized, irreversible lesions may be already present. (2) In some cases, the causative drug involved in acute hepatitis is not recognized and its administration is continued. (3) In other cases, the causative drug has been withdrawn but is later read-ministered before complete recovery. (4) In a few cases, the process leading to liver injury persists despite withdrawal of the offending drug. This has been observed with amiodarone [70] and perhexiline [65] which exhibit extensive tissue storage and are slowly released into the systemic circulation. It may also occur with drugs such as tienilic acid, which trig-gers an autoimmune response against normal hepatocyte constituents [5].

Prolonged necrosis may lead to subacute hepatitis, chronic hepati-tis, and cirrhosis. The agents mainly responsible for causing subacute hepatitis, chronic hepatitis, and cirrhosis are amiodarone iproniazid, methotrexate, methyldopa, nitrofurantoin, papaverine, and vitamin A (Table 3). Clometacin, tienilic acid, and perhexilline have been with-drawn from pharmaceutical markets because of fatal cirrhosis.

Table 3. Main drugs responsible for subacute hepatitis, chronic hepatitis, or cirrhosis (adapted from [66, 85, 90])

Acetohexamide	Metahexamide
Amiodarone	Methotrexate
Amodiaquine	Methyldopa
Aspirin	Nitrofurantoin
Benzarone	Papaverine
Busulfan	Paracetamol
Chlorambucil	Perhexiline
Clometacin	Propylthiouracil
Dantrolene	Suloctidil
Frentizole	Tienilic acid
Glafenine	Urethane
Halothane	Valproic acid
Iproniazid	Vitamin A
Isoniazid	

2.2.1 Clinicopathological Features

2.2.1.1 Subacute Hepatitis [90].
Clinical and biochemical manifestations persist or even worsen within a few weeks or months following the onset of jaundice. In some cases, ascites, encephalopathy, hypoalbuminemia, and hypoprothrombinemia develop. Histologically, subacute hepatitis is characterized by lesions at different stages of evolution. Acute lesions consist of lobular necrosis with inflammatory infiltration such as seen in acute hepatitis. Secondary lesions consist of bridging necrosis, that is necrosis and subsequent cell dropout thereby linking two portal tracts together or a portal tract and a central vein. Late lesions are suggestive of a chronic process, with portal fibrosis and inflammatory infiltration of portal tracts and, in some cases, nodules of regeneration. Subacute

hepatitis occurs mainly when the causative drug has been readminis-
tered before complete recovery or when it has been continued despite
overt liver injury.

2.2.1.2 Chronic Hepatitis [66]. Symptoms are generally absent or nonspecific over a long period of time. Serum aminotransferases are
increased as is the serum γ-globulin level. Histologic findings consist of
periportal hepatocyte necrosis (piecemeal necrosis) and portal
inflammation and fibrosis, both of which may extend into the peripheral
parenchyma.

2.2.1.3 Cirrhosis. The clinical manifestations of *cirrhosis* are extremely
variable. It may be recognized fortuitously or may be revealed by the
presence of jaundice, ascites, hepatic encephalopathy, hepatomegaly, or
complications of portal hypertension. Serum aminotransferase activity
often moderately increases. Hypoalbuminemia and hypoprothrombinemia are common. Histologically, cirrhosis is characterized by a destruction of lobular architecture, extensive fibrosis, and nodules of regeneration. These lesions may be associated with those of subacute or chronic
hepatitis.

2.2.2 Immunological Disorders

The three liver lesions described above are frequently associated with
immunological disorders, in particular serum autoantibodies [25]. Nonspecific antibodies such as anti-nuclear or anti-smooth muscle antibodies are observed with several drugs, including clometacin, methyldopa,
and papaverine [25]. In contrast, other serum autoantibodies appear to
be more specific and may be used as diagnostic markers of drug-induced
liver injury: anti-LKM2 with tienilic acid [5], anti-LM with dihydralazine [10], type 6 anti-mitochondrial antibodies and iproniazid [25].

2.3 Granulomatous Hepatitis

Pathological changes consist of numerous noncaseating granulomas distributed throughout lobular areas and portal tracts. Granulomas are
made up of small foci of epithelioid cells and occasionally contain eosinophils or giant cells. Hepatic granulomas may be associated with other
liver lesions such as hepatocellular necrosis or cholestasis. Granulomatous hepatitis may be completely asymptomatic, characterized only by
biological changes. Jaundice, pruritus, and hepatomegaly may be present either when granulomas are numerous or in the presence of associated liver lesions. Serum AP and γ-glutamyltransferase activities are frequently increased. Granulomatous hepatitis may be associated with

hypersensitivity manifestations. The diagnosis relies upon histologic examination. The main drugs responsible for granulomatous hepatitis are allopurinol, carbamazepine, phenylbutazone, quinidine, hydralazine, dapsone, gold salts, nitrofurantoin, and sulfonamides [30, 54]. Liver disorders disappear after discontinuation of the offending treatment.

2.4 Steatosis

Steatosis is characterized by the accumulation of lipids,mostly triglycerides, in hepatocytes. Two types may be distinguished, macrovacuolar and microvesicular steatosis, exhibiting different clinical and prognostic features [22, 90].

2.4.1 Macrovacuolar Steatosis

This form is characterized by the presence of a single large droplet of fat in hepatocytes displacing the nucleus to the periphery of the cell. Mild or moderate macrovacuolar steatosis remains asymptomatic. When lesions are extensive, jaundice, abdominal pain, and hepatomegaly may be present. Serum aminotransferase and γ-glutamyltransferase activities are moderately increased. Macrovacuolar steatosis exhibits a very good prognosis. However, it may be associated with more severe liver lesions such as hepatocellular necrosis. The main causative drugs are corticosteroids, methotrexate, and asparaginase [22, 90].

2.4.2 Microvesicular Steatosis

This form contrasts point by point to with macrovacuolar steatosis. The lesion is similar to that seen in Reye's syndrome and consists of numerous small lipid droplets without displacement of the hepatocyte nucleus. Microvesicular steatosis may be isolated, as with tetracycline, or associated with liver cell necrosis, as with pirprofen or valproic acid. Moderate microvesicular steatosis may be asymptomatic or only revealed by asthenia, nausea, or vomiting. Serum aminotransferase activities and bilirubin are moderately increased. When extensive, microvesicular steatosis may lead to hepatic failure, hypoglycemia, and coma with a fatal course. Renal failure and pancreatitis may also be present, contributing to the poor prognosis. The main causative drugs are cycline derivatives given intravenously at high doses [90], valproic acid, salicylates and less frequently, NSAIDS from the 2-arylpropionic acid family (pirprofen, ketoprofen, ibuprofen) [8], and amineptine [22]. Microvesicular steatosis is probably related to drug-induced inhibition of mitochondrial β-oxidation of fatty acids [9, 23].

2.5 Phospholipidosis and Alcohol-Induced Type Liver Lesions

2.5.1 Phospholipidosis

Liver phospholipidosis is characterized by the accumulation of phospholipids within hepatocyte lysosomes [51]. It has been observed with three anti-anginal drugs: amiodarone [47, 70, 79], perhexiline maleate [65], and 4,4-diethylaminoethoxyhexestrol [15]. These drugs are cationic amphophilic compounds with a lipophil moiety and ionizable nitrogen [51]. These properties promote accumulation of the drugs within liver cell lysosomes. As a consequence, lysosomal phospholipases may be inhibited, which results in accumulation of phospholipids [51]. Due to extensive tissue storage leading to slow elimination, the drugs may be detectable in plasma several weeks or months after discontinuation of the treatment [79]. Isolated liver phospholipidosis exhibits no clinical consequence. The diagnosis relies upon electron microscopic examination showing lamellar or pseudomyelinic figures in lysosomes.

2.5.2 Alcohol-Induced Type Lesions

Generally, these lesions occur in patients who have received long-term treatment [47, 65, 70, 79]. Their frequency seems to be correlated with the cumulative dose. The disease usually develops insidiously. It may be revealed by asthenia, hepatomegaly, or a moderate increase in aminotransferases, or, at late stage, by complications of cirrhosis. Histologic examination shows lesions simulating acute alcoholic hepatitis, including acidophil necrosis, Mallory's bodies, neutrophil infiltration, and steatosis in lobular areas; portal fibrosis or cirrhosis may be associated. Discontinuation of the treatment is usually followed by progressive regression of liver disorders. In some cases, however, the condition of the liver further deteriorates and the disorder may be fatal, probably because of protracted release of the drug into the systemic circulation from tissue storage sites. Perhexiline hepatotoxicity is strongly related to a genetic deficiency in hepatic cytochrome P-450 2D6, which causes accumulation of the drug in the liver [58]. The frequency of this deficiency in most populations, particularly in Europe, is about 7 %–10 %. Occasionally, alcohol-induced type liver injury phospholipidosis may also be observed after administration of nifedipine [3] and diltiazem [4].

2.6 Vascular Diseases of the Liver

Drug reactions make up an important cause of vascular diseases of the liver [87, 89] (Table 4). The most significant ones are described below.

2.6.1 Perisinusoidal Fibrosis

This lesion results from the accumulation of collagen within Disse's space. Perisinusoidal fibrosis may remain asymptomatic or be revealed by hepatomegaly or venous portal hypertension. Chronic hypervitaminosis A is the main cause of this disorder. The accumulation of vitamin A may be demonstrated by light and electron microscopy showing Ito cell hyperplasia. Liver vitamin A concentration is highly increased. Portal fibrosis or even cirrhosis may occur if vitamin A administration is protracted. Other causative agents are azathioprine, 6-mercaptopurine, methotrexate, and arsenic derivatives [87, 89].

2.6.2 Peliosis Hepatis

Peliosis hepatis is histologically characterized by blood-filled cavities, bordered by hepatocytes, randomly distributed throughout the liver. In most cases, peliosis hepatis is asymptomatic and liver tests are normal or only moderately disturbed. In some cases, the condition may be revealed by hepatomegaly, jaundice, portal hypertension, and even hepatic failure or hemoperitoneum. The main causative agents are 17-α-alkylated anabolic-androgenic steroids [29], azathioprine [14], 6-thioguanine [38] and arsenic derivatives [87, 89]. The role of oral contraceptives remains controversial.

2.6.3 Venoocclusive Disease

This disease is characterized by nonthrombotic obstruction of small centrilobular veins resulting in congestion and liver cell necrosis in the centrilobular area. The clinical presentation of venoocclusive disease may be acute or chronic. The acute form is characterized by the prompt onset of abdominal pain and ascites and may evolve either to recovery or to fatal hepatic failure. The disease may also develop insidiously, leading to extensive central fibrosis and eventually to cirrhosis. Venoocclusive disease was initially observed after ingestion of medicinal plants used for decoctions and infusions and containing pyrrolizidine alkaloids. Now, the disease mainly occurs in patients treated with irradiation and chemotherapy, as required for preparation of bone marrow transplantation [87, 89]. It has also been observed with some drugs (Table 4).

Table 4. Drugs responsible for vascular lesions of the liver (adapted from [87, 89])

Thrombosis of portal vein and its main branches
    Oral contraceptives
    Arsenic derivatives
	Venoocclusive disease
	    Pyrrolizidine alkaloids
	    Urethane
	    Azathioprine
	    6-Thioguanine
	    6-Mercaptopurine
	    Dacarbazine
	    Doxorubicin[a]
	    Mitomycin[a]
	    Vincristine[a]
	    Indicine N-oxide[a]
	    Carmustine (BCNU)[a]
	    Vitamin E (intravenous)[a]
	    Progestins[a]
	    Cysteamine[a]

Lesions of hepatic artery and its branches
    Arterial intimal hyperplasia
        Oral contraceptives
    Angiitis
        Methamphetamine[a]	

Perisinusoidal fibrosis
    Vitamin A
    Azathioprine
    6-Mercaptopurine
    Methotrexate
    Arsenic derivatives
    Thorium dioxide
    Urethane[a]	

	Budd-Chiari syndrome
	    Oral contraceptives
	    Dacarbazine
	    Doxorubicin
	    Vincristine
	    Cyclosphosphamide

Sinusoidal dilation
    Oral contraceptives
    Azathioprine
    Chenodeoxycholic acid[a]	

Peliosis hepatis
    Anabolic-androgenic steroids
    Azathioprine
    Arsenic derivatives
    Thorium dioxide
    Oral contraceptives[a]
    Corticosteroids[a]
    Medroxyprogesterone[a]
    Tamoxifen[a]
    Estrone sulfate[a]
	Lesions possibly related to vascular injury
	    Hepatoportal sclerosis
	        Vitamin A
	        Azathioprine
	        Methotrexate
	        Arsenic derivatives
	        Thorium dioxide
	    Nodular regenerative hyperplasia
	        Azathioprine
	        Anabolic-androgenic steroids[a]
	        Oral contraceptives[a]
	        Corticosteroids[a]

[a] Drugs for which the causal relationship should be confirmed.

2.6.4 Budd-Chiari Syndrome

Budd-Chiari syndrome is characterized by the obstruction of large hepatic veins resulting in hepatic congestion and liver cell necrosis. The severity of the syndrome varies with the site and extent of thrombosis. The clinical presentation may be acute, with abdominal pain or ascites, or chronic, mimicking decompensated cirrhosis [87, 89]. The spigalian lobe, spared by the disease, is hypertrophic. The risk of developing Budd-Chiari syndrome is 2.5-fold higher in oral contraceptive users. Oral contraceptives may act mainly by exacerbating an underlying thrombogenic condition, in particular, a latent myeloproliferative disease [87]. Budd-Chiari syndrome has also been observed in patients receiving some anticancer drugs (Table 4).

2.7 Hepatic Tumors

2.7.1 Hepatocellular Adenoma

Hepatocellular adenoma is a benign tumor consisting of normal, tightly packed hepatocyte plates without a portal tract or centrilobular vein. Oral contraceptive users are more susceptible to the development of hepatic adenomas [2, 86]. This effect is mainly caused by the estrogenic component of the drug. The incidence of adenoma appears to be time- and probably also dose-dependent. The relative risk has been described as being slightly increased between 1 and 3 years of oral contraceptive use, 116-fold at 5 years, and more than 500-fold after 7 years [74]. The estimated incidence was 1 per million in females taking no oral contraceptives compared to 34 per million in users of oral contraceptives. It is noteworthy, however, that the amount of estrogens present in the new oral contraceptives used during the last decade is much lower. Therefore, the incidence of adenoma might have also decreased. This point deserves new epidemiological studies. The tumor is generally asymptomatic and is often discovered by ultrasonography. Less frequently, it is revealed by hepatomegaly, abdominal pain, or by intraperitoneal or intratumoral bleeding. These complications occur mostly with large tumors and may be promoted by oral contraceptive intake. The discontinuation of oral contraceptives is occasionally followed by a slow reduction of tumor size. Adenoma can recur following readministration of oral contraceptives or pregnancy. The degeneration of oral contraceptive-induced adenoma into hepatocellular carcinoma remains controversial [86].

The risk of developing a hepatic adenoma is also increased by prolonged administration of 17-α-alkylated anabolic-androgenic steroids [29]. Adenoma caused by these agents may evolve to hepatocellular carcinoma. Exceptional cases of adenoma have also been observed after administration of clomiphene and norethisterone [86].

2.7.2 Hepatocellular Carcinoma

The risk of developing hepatocellular carcinoma appears to be increased by prolonged administration of anabolic-androgenic steroids [2, 29]. The relative risk might be increased from 7 to 20 times in women age 20–50 years taking oral contraceptives for at least 8 years. Hepatocellular carcinoma related to anabolic-androgenic steroids and oral contraceptives exhibits features other than those seen in hepatocellular carcinoma complicating cirrhosis [29]: It occurs mainly in relatively young subjects; the α-fetoprotein level is generally normal [29]; metastasis is uncommon; nontumoral liver is normal. Hepatocellular carcinoma induced by anabolic-androgenic steroids sometimes recedes after drug discontinuation. The role of steroids in the incidence of fibrolamellar carcinoma is still unknown.

2.7.3 Angiosarcoma

This is an uncommon malignant tumor developed from endothelial cells present in sinusoids. It has been observed after administration of some drugs including arsenic derivatives, anabolic-androgenic steroids, oral contraceptives, and phenelzine [2].

2.7.4 Cholangiocarcinoma

This is a malignant tumor made up of cells resembling biliary epithelial cells. The tumor has been observed in subjects exposed to thorium dioxide and, occasionally, in patients receiving long-term anabolic-androgenic steroid therapy, oral contraceptive, methyldopa or methotrexate. The causal relationship between these drugs and this tumor, however, remains to be confirmed [2].

3 Biliary Tract Injuries

The toxicity of drugs to the biliary tract has been only recently recognized. The number of involved drugs (about 50) is much lower than for drug-induced hepatotoxicity [40].

3.1 Acute Injuries Involving Small Bile Ducts

These correspond to acute cholangiolitis and cholangitis. Cholangiolitis refers to inflammation of the ductules and is characterized by inflammatory infiltration by polymorphonuclear leukocytes in and around the ductules and by edema and ductular proliferation. Cholangitis refers to edema and acute inflammatory infiltration in and around portal bile ducts. Both lesions are frequently associated with a predominance of cholangitis. Severe lesions are marked by bile duct dilatation and necrosis of biliary epithelial cells. Cholangiolitis and cholangitis may be isolated [39] or associated with hepatocyte lesions such as necrosis or granuloma [46]. In the latter case it may be difficult to determine the relative contribution of biliary and hepatic lesions to the symptoms and the underlying biological disorder. Manifestations are similar to those of acute cholestatic hepatitis and can simulate acute biliary obstruction by associating abdominal pain and high grade fever preceding jaundice [39, 46]. The association with hypersensitivity manifestations (blood hypereosinophilia, skin rash) is frequent and suggests a drug reaction. In most cases, recovery occurs rapidly after discontinuation of the causative treatment. Uncommonly, however, the acute episode may be followed by chronic cholangitis [13, 61] (see below).

Albeit not clearly elucidated, the mechanisms leading to acute injuries of small bile ducts seem to involve immunoallergic phenomena [37, 90]. The main causative drugs are chlorpromazine, allopurinol, carbamazepine, and phenytoin (Table 5).

3.2 Chronic Injuries Involving Small Intrahepatic Bile Ducts

Compared to drug-induced acute hepatitis or acute cholangitis, only a minority of patients develops prolonged cholestasis [37, 90]. This syndrome may be defined by the persistence of jaundice for more than 6 months or the persistence of biochemical disorders consistent with anicteric cholestasis, i.e., high AP and γ-glutamyltransferase activities, for more than 1 year despite withdrawal of the causative drug and in the absence of a previous history of chronic liver and biliary tract disease [37]. This definition excludes cases in which the initial acute drug-induced injury is not well characterized and those in which asymptomatic preexisting hepatic or biliary disease cannot be eliminated. This syndrome has been observed with about 30 drugs, mainly chlorpromazine and other phenothiazine derivatives [28, 90], ajmaline [42], arsenic derivatives [83] and tricyclic antidepressants [33] (Table 6).

Table 5. Main drugs responsible for acute lesions of small bile ducts (acute cholangiolitis and cholangitis) (adapted from [40])

Ajmaline	Diazepam
Amitriptyline	Difetarsone (arsenic derivative)
Amoxicillin-clavulanic acid	Glibenclamide
Ampicillin	Interleukin-2
Allopurinol	Penicillamine
Azathioprine	Phenytoin
Barbiturates	Hydralazine
Carbamazepine	Metahexamide
Chlorothiazide	Methyltestosterone
Chlorpromazine	Troleandomycin
Chlorpropamide	Gold salts
Clometacin	Sulindac

Table 6. Drugs responsible for chronic lesions of small bile ducts (chronic cholangitis) (adapted from [40])

Aceprometazine (+ meprobamate)	Haloperidol
Ajmaline	Imipramine
Amitriptyline	Methyltestosterone
Ampicillin	Norandrostenolone cyclohexypropionate
Arsenic derivatives	Phenytoin
Barbiturates	Prochlorperazine
Carbamazepine	Thiabendazole
Carbutamide	Tiopronin
Chlorpromazine	Tolbutamide
Cimetidine	Trimethoprim-sulfamethoxazole
Cyproheptadine	(cotrimoxazole)
Erythromycin	Troleandomycin
Flucloxacillin	Xenolamine

For chlorpromazine and ajmaline, the frequency of chronic cholangitis has been estimated to be about 7 % – 10 % of patients with acute hepatitis or cholangitis [37, 90]. Two types of disease have been characterized according to severity [37, 90].

The major form, observed in about 25 % patients, is characterized by the persistence or even worsening of jaundice and pruritus after initial injury. Xanthomata and xanthelasma, malabsorption syndrome, splenomegaly, and hepatomegaly may also be seen in the most severe cases. Biochemical disorders include high serum AP and γ-glutamyltransferase activities and high bile acid concentration, hyperbilirubinemia (constant in this form), and hypercholesterolemia. Serum aminotransferases are normal or moderately increased. The pathological features resemble those of primary biliary cirrhosis. Portal tracts lesions are prominent, including the disappearance of interlobular bile ducts, ductular proliferation, and moderate and polymorphous inflammatory infiltration containing polymorphonuclear cells [13]. Lobular lesions include cholestasis and, sometimes, pseudoxanthomatous degeneration or necrosis of periportal hepatocytes. Portal fibrosis is generally absent or moderate [28]. The spontaneous course of the disease is generally good, in contrast with primary biliary cirrhosis. In most patients, jaundice finally subsides, sometimes several years after the onset of the disease and AP and γ-glutamyltransferase activities tend to decrease slowly [37, 90]. In one patient, these disorders were still present 14 years after the onset of the disease. In about 25 % of patients, jaundice persists and secondary biliary cirrhosis develops (chlorpromazine, ajmaline, flucloxacillin, imipramine, thiabendazole, tiopronine) [40, 90]. A fatal course has been observed with carbutamide, tolbutamide, chlorpromazine, methyltestosterone, and thiabendazole [37, 90]. Liver transplantation should be proposed in patients with irreversible lesions with signs of severity.

The minor form, observed in about 75 % of patients, is characterized by the disappearance of jaundice and pruritus in less than 3 months [37, 90]. Then, liver dysfunction generally becomes asymptomatic and consists of high AP and γ-glutamyltransferase activities. The lesions are characterized histologically by partial disappearance of small bile ducts, mild or moderate portal inflammation, and mild or no fibrosis. These liver disorders progressively decrease and can disappear several years after the onset of the disease [37].

The mechanism of drug-induced chronic cholangitis is unknown. It is presently believed to involve autoimmune phenomena. However, attempts to improve the course of the disease by corticosteroid therapy have been unsuccessful [21]. The treatment is mainly symptomatic and consists of relieving pruritus and avoiding malabsorption.

3.3 Acute and Chronic Injuries Involving Large Intra- and Extrahepatic Bile Ducts

Two types can be distinguished according to the physiopathological mechanism involved.

3.3.1 Ischemic Cholangitis

This type mainly occurs after chemotherapy and, less frequently, after intraarterial hepatic embolization for the treatment of liver metastasis or hepatocarcinoma [1, 16, 31].

3.3.1.1 Chemotherapy. Sclerosing cholangitis is a major and late complication of intraarterial hepatic infusion of floxuridine (FUDR) in patients with liver metastasis from colorectal carcinoma. This complication is frequent (5 %–29 % treated subjects) and is characterized by progressive cholestasis. Cholangiography reveals segmental structures generally affecting both intra- and extrahepatic bile ducts [16, 31]. Strictures almost always involve the confluence of hepatic ducts and spare the distal common bile duct, in contrast to primary sclerosing cholangitis. Exceptionally, the disease may mimic Caroli's disease [69]. Bile duct strictures are reversible in some patients. The disease may result from bile duct ischemia caused by lesion of arterioles supplying the upper part of the common bile duct. Arterial lesions may also be provoked by the surgery required for setting the infusion pump in the hepatic artery and/or by toxic effects of FUDR. Intraarterial infusion of dexamethasone together with FUDR might contribute to preventing this complication [62].

Other injurious chemotherapy agents are 5-fluorouracil associated or not with streptozotocin, mitomycin, and the combination mitomycin-doxorubicin [40].

3.3.1.2 Embolization. Treatment of hepatocarcinoma by embolization may lead to ischemic cholangitis [52].

3.3.2 Caustic Cholangitis

Agents used during surgery for sterilizing hydatid cysts can produce toxic biliary lesions when cysts communicate with the biliary tract. This may result in sclerosing cholangitis. Causative compounds are 20 % hypertonic saline and 2 % formol [6].

3.4 Drug-Induced Biliary Lithiasis

Some drugs can promote the formation of cholesterol or bilirubin gallstones or may themselves comprise part of the stone [40].

3.4.1 Cholesterol Gallstones

The risk of developing cholesterol gallstones is increased by long-term administration of oral contraceptives [12], medroxyprogesterone [55], clofibrate [82], octreotide [17, 53], and perharps ciclosporin [80]. Gallstone formation appears to be mainly related to bile cholesterol supersaturation for oral contraceptives and clofibrate and to bile stasis for octreotide and medroxyprogesterone.

3.4.2 Bilirubin Gallstones

All drugs responsible for hemolysis may thereby lead to pigment lithiasis.

3.4.3 Drug-Induced Lithiasis

The development of sludge or stones in the gallbladder has been frequently observed in subjects treated with large doses of ceftriaxone, a third-generation cephalosporin, intravenously [24, 72, 76]. Biliary concretions develop within 1–2 weeks, sometimes causing symptoms. After cessation of ceftriaxone treatment, complete resolution occurs on average within 2 weeks. The formation of these stones results from the precipitation of calcium-ceftriaxone salts within the gallbladder. Similarly, precipitation of glafenine in the biliary tract may rarely lead to concretions responsible for bile duct obstruction in patients receiving protracted treatment [11, 57].

3.5 Acalculous Cholecystitis

Intraarterial hepatic chemotherapy for liver metastasis from colorectal carcinoma is followed by cholecystitis in 30 % of patients [75]. Consequently, preventive cholecystectomy has been proposed by some authors to avoid this complication.

Similarly cholecystitis may also occur after embolization with gelatin powder or Lipiodol (iodized oil) [52, 88]. The existence of allergic cholecystitis has been recently suggested; potential offending drugs are ampicillin and erythromycin [64].

Acalculous cholecystitis has sometimes been observed after lysophosphatidylcholine administration [59].

4 Conclusions

Drug reactions may reproduce almost all acute and chronic diseases of the liver and biliary tract. The diagnosis is frequently difficult and mainly relies upon exclusion criteria. Hypersensitivity manifestations are often present in acute hepatitis and cholangitis affecting some bile ducts, which facilitates the diagnosis and suggests an immunoallergic mechanism. In all cases, treatment essentially consists of discontinuing administration of the offending drug.

Acknowledgements. We thank Josette Viala and Stéphanie Larrey for preparation of the manuscript.

References

1. Anderson SD, Nolley HC, Berland LL, Van Dyke JA, Stanley R (1986) Causes of jaundice during hepatic artery infusion chemotherapy. Radiology 161: 439–442
2. Anthony PP (1988) Liver tumours. Bailliere's Clin Gastroenterol 2: 501–522
3. Babany G, Uzzan F, Larrey D, Degott C, Bourgeois C, René E, Vissuzaine C, Erlinger S, Benhamou JP (1989) Alcoholic-like liver lesions induced by nifedipine. J Hepatol 9: 252–255
4. Beaugrand M, Denis J, Callard P (1987) Tous les inhibiteurs calciques peuvent-ils entraîner des lésions d'hépatite alcoolique? Gastroenterol Clin Biol 10: 76
5. Beaune PH, Dansette PM, Mansuy D et al. (1987) Human anti-endoplasmic reticulum autoantibodies appearing in a drug-induced hepatitis are directed against a human liver cytochrome P-450 that hydroxylates the drug. Proc Nat Acad Sci USA 84: 551–555
6. Belghiti J, Benhamou JP, Houry S, Grenier P, Huguier M, Fekete F (1986) Caustic sclerosing cholangitis. A complication of the surgical treatment of hydatid disease of the liver. Arch Surg 121: 1162–1165
7. Benichou C and an international group of experts (1990) Criteria of drug-induced liver disorders. J Hepatol 11: 272–276

8. Biour M, Poupon R, Grange JD, Chazouilleres O, Levy VG, Bodin F, Cheymol G (1991) Hépatotoxicité des médicaments. Mise à jour du fichier bibliographique des atteintes hépatiques et des médicaments responsables. Gastroenterol Clin Biol 15: 64–78

9. Bjorge SM, Baillie TA (1985) Inhibition of medium-chain fatty acid β-oxidation in vitro by valproic acid and its unsaturated metabolite, 2-n-propyl-4-pentenoic acid. Biochem Biophys Res Com 132: 245–252

10. Bourdi M, Larrey D, Nataf J, Bernuau J, Pessayre D, Iwasaki M, Guengerich FP, Beaune PH (1990) Anti-liver endoplasmic reticulum auto-antibodies are directed against human cytochrome P-450 IA2. A specific marker of dihydralazine-induced hepatitis. J Clin Invest 85: 1967–1973

11. Daudon M, Reveillaud RJ, Bigorie B (1988) Lithiase médicamenteuse du cholédoque. Presse Med 17: 869

12. Davion T, Capron JP (1991) Epidémiologie et facteurs de risque de la lithiase biliaire. In: Erlinger S, éd. La lithiase biliaire. Paris: Doin: 1–15

13. Degott C, Feldmann G, Larrey D, Durand-Schneider AM, Grange D, Machayekhi JP, Moreau A, Potet F, Benhamou JP (1992 Drug-induced prolonged cholestasis in adults: a histological semiquantitative study demonstrating progressive ductopenia. Hepatology 15: 244–251

14. Degott C, Rueff B, Kreis H, Duboust A, Potet F, Benhamou JP (1978) Peliosis hepatis in recipients of renal transplants. Gut 19: 748–753

15. De La Inglesia FA, Feuer G, Takada A, Matsuda Y (1974) Morphologic studies on secondary phospholipidosis in humans. Lab Invest 4: 539–549

16. Dikengil A, Siskind BN, Morse SS, Swedlund A, Bober-Sorcinelli KE, Burrel MI (1986) Sclerosing cholangitis from intra-arterial floxuridine. J Clin Gastroenterol 8: 690–693

17. Dowling RH, Hussaini SH, Murphy GM, Besser GM, Wass JAH (1992) Gallstones during octreotide therapy. Metabolism 41: 22–33

18. Dutertre JP, Bastides F, Jonville AP, De Muret A, Sonneville A, Larrey D, Autret E (1991) Microvesicular steatosis after ketoprofen administration. Eur J Gastroenterol Hepatol 3: 953–954

19. Eade OE, Grice D, Krawitt EL et al. (1981) HLA A and B locus antigens in patients with unexplained hepatitis following halothane anaesthesia. Tissue Antigens 17: 428–432

20. Farrell G, Prendergast D, Murray M (1985) Halothane hepatitis. Detection of a constitutional susceptibility factor. N Engl J Med 313: 1310–1314

21. Forbes GM, Jeffrey GP, Shilkin KB, Reed WD (1992) Carbamazepine hepatotoxicity: another cause of the vanishing bile duct syndrome. Gastroenterology 102: 1385–1388

22. Freneaux E, Larrey D, Pessayre D (1988) Stéatoses hépatiques médicamenteuses à triglycérides. Rev Fr Gastroenterol 240: 873–884

23. Geneve J, Hayat-Bonan B, Degott C, Letteron P, Freneaux E, Le Dinh T, Larrey D, Pessayre D (1987) Inhibition of mitochondrial β-oxidation of fatty acids by pirprofen. Role in microvesicular steatosis due to this nonsteroidal anti-inflammatory drug. J Pharmacol Exp Ther 242: 1133–1137

24. Heim-Duthoy KL, Caperton EM, Pollock R, Matzke GR, Enthoven D, Peterson PK (1990) Apparent biliary pseudolithiasis during ceftriaxone therapy. Antimicrob Agents Chemother 34: 1146–1149

25. Homberg JC, Abuaf N, Helmy-Khalil S, Biour M, Poupon R, Islam S, Darnis F, Levy VG, Opolon P, Beaugrand M, Toulet J, Danan G, Benhamou JP (1985) Drug-induced hepatitis associated with anticytoplasmic organelle autoantibodies. Hepatology 5: 722–727

26. Horsmans Y, Lannes D, Pessayre D, Larrey D. (1991) Possible relationship between Atrium-induced hepatotoxicity and the genetic polymorphism in mephenytoin oxidation. Gastroenterology 100: A 828

27. Horsmans Y, Larrey D, Pessayre D, Benhamou JP (1990) Hépatotoxité des médicaments anti-infectieux. Première partie: Les antibiotiques antibactériens. Gastroenterol Clin Biol 14: 911–918
28. Ishak KG, Irey NS (1972) Hepatic injury associated with the phenothiazines. Clinico-pathologic and follow-up study of 36 patients. Arch Pathol 93: 283–304
29. Ishak KG, Zimmermann HJ (1987) Hepatotoxic effects of the anabolic-androgenic steroids. Semin Liver Dis 7: 230–236
30. Ishak KG, Zimmermann HJ (1988) Drug-induced and toxic granulomatous hepatitis. Baillere's clin gastroenterol 2: 463–480
31. Kemeny N, Daly J, Reichman B, Geller N, Botet J, Oderman P (1987) Intrahepatic or systemic infusion of fluorodeoxyuridine in patients with liver metastases from colorectal carcinoma. A randomized trial. Ann Intern Med 107: 459–465
32. Larrey D, Amouyal G, Danan G, Degott C, Pessayre D, Benhamou JP (1987) Prolonged cholestasis after troleandomycin-induced acute hepatitis. J Hepatol 4: 327–329
33. Larrey D, Amouyal G, Pessayre D, Degott C, Danne O, Machayekhi JP, Feldmann G, Benhamou JP (1988) Amitriptyline-induced prolonged cholestasis. Gastroenterology 94: 200–203
34. Larrey D, Babany G, Bernuau J, Andrieux J, Degott C, Pessayre D, Benhamou JP. (1990) Fulminant hepatitis after lisinopril administration. Gastroenterology 99: 1832–1833
35. Larrey D, Berson A, Habersetzer F, Tinel M, Castot A, Babany G, Lettéron P, Freneaux E, Loeper J, Dansette P, Pessayre D (1989) Genetic predisposition to drug hepatotoxicity. Role in hepatitis caused by amineptine, a tricyclic antidepressant. Hepatology 10: 168–173
36. Larrey D, Castot A, Pessayre D, Merigot P, Machayekhi JP, Feldmann G, Lenoir A, Rueff B, Benhamou JP (1986) Amodiaquine-induced hepatitis. A report of seven cases. Ann Intern Med 104: 801–803
37. Larrey D, Erlinger S (1988) Drug-induced cholestasis. Bailliere's Clinical Gastroenterol 2: 423–452
38. Larrey D, Freneaux E, Berson A, Babany G, Degott C, Valla D, Pessayre D, Benhamou JP (1988) Peliosis hepatis induced by 6-thioguanine administration. Gut 29: 1265–1269
39. Larrey D, Hadengue A, Pessayre D, Choudat L, Degott C, Benhamou JP (1987) Carbamazepine-induced acute cholangitis. Dig Dis Sci 32: 554–557
40. Larrey D, Michel H (1993) Pathologie biliaire dûe aux médicaments. Gastroenterol clin biol (in press)
41. Larrey D, Pessayre D (1988) Genetic factors in hepatotoxicity. In: Liver cells and drugs. Ed Guillouzo A, Libbey J, London 164: 143–152
42. Larrey D, Pessayre D, Duhamel G, Casier A, Degott C, Feldmann G, Erlinger S, Benhamou JP (1986) Prolonged cholestasis after ajmaline-induced acute hepatitis. J Hepatol 2: 81–87
43. Larrey D, Rueff B, Pessayre D, Danan G, Algard M, Geneve J, Benhamou JP (1986) Cross hepatotoxicity between tricyclic antidepressants. Gut 27: 726–727
44. Larrey D, Vial T, Micaleff A, Babany G, Morichau-Beauchant M, Michel H, Benhamou JP (1992) Hepatitis associated with amoxycillin-clavulanic acid combination report of 15 cases. Gut 33: 368-371
45. Larrey D, Vial T, Pauwels A, Castot A, Biour M, David M, Michel H (1992) Hepatitis after germander (Teucrium chamaedrys) administration: another instance of herbal medicine hepatotoxicity. Ann Intern Med 117: 129–132
46. Levy M, Goodman M, Van Dyne BJ, Hatton S (1981) Granulomatous hepatitis secondary to carbamazepine. Ann Intern Med 95: 64–65
47. Lewis JH, Ranard RC, Caruso A, Jackson LK, Mullick F, Ishak KG, Seeff LB, Zimmermann HJ (1989) Amiodarone hepatotoxicity: prevalence and clinico-pathologic correlations among 104 patients. Hepatology 9: 679–685

48. Loeper J, Descatoire V, Amouyal G, Lettéron P, Larrey D, Pessayre D (1989) Presence of covalently bound metabolites on rat hepatocyte plasma membrane proteins after administration of isaxonine, a drug leading to immunoallergic hepatitis in man. Hepatology 9: 675–678
49. Loeper J, Descatoire V, Maurice M, Beaune P, Feldmann G, Larrey D, Pessayre D (1990) Presence of functional cytochrome P-450 on isolated rat hepatocyte plasma membrane. Hepatology 11: 850–858
50. Ludwig J, Kim CH, Wiesner RH, Krom RAF (1989) Floxuridine-induced sclerosing cholangitis: an ischemic cholangiopathy? Hepatology 9: 215–218
51. Lüllmann H, Lüllmann-Rauch R, Wassermann O (1975) Drug-induced phospholipidoses. CRC Critical Rev Toxicol 4: 185–242
52. Makuuchi M, Sukigara M, Mori T, Kobayashi J, Yamazaki S, Hasegawa H (1985) Bile duct necrosis: compilation of transcatheter hepatic arterial embolization. Radiology 156: 331–334
53. McKnight JA, McCance DR, Atkinson AB, Crothers JG (1989) Changes in glucose tolerance and development of gallstones during high dose treatment with octreotide for acromegaly. Br Med J 299: 1162–1163
54. McMaster KR, Hennigar GG (1981) Drug-induced granulomatous hepatitis. Lab Invest 44: 61–73
55. Meyer WJ, Wiener I, Emory LE, Cole CM, Isenberg N, Fagan CJ et al. (1992) Cholelithiasis associated with medroxyprogesterone acetate therapy in men. Res Comm Chem Pathol Pharmacol 75: 69–84
56. Miguet JP, Vuitton D, Allemand H et al. (1980) Une épidémie d'ictères dus à l'association troléandomycine-contraceptifs oraux. Gastroenterol Clin Biol 4: 420–424
57. Moesch C, Gainant A, Sautereau D (1988) Lithiase biliaire de glafénine. Identification par spectrophotométrie infrarouge. Gastroenterol Clin Biol 12: 387–389
58. Morgan MY, Reshef R, Shah RR, Oates NS, Smith RL, Sherlock S (1984) Impaired oxidation of debrisoquine in patients with perhexiline liver injury. Gut 1057–1064
59. Neiderhiser DH (1986) Acute acalculous cholecystitis induced by lysophosphatidylcholine. Am J Pathol 124: 559–563
60. Neuberger, J, Forman D, Doll R, Williams R (1986) Oral contraceptives and hepatocellular carcinoma. Br Med J 292: 1355-1357
61. Pagliaro L, Campesi G, Aguglia F (1969) Barbiturate jaundice. Report of a case due to a barbital-containing drug, with positive rechallenge to phenobarbital. Gastroenterology 56: 938–943
62. Paquette P, Campos LT, Flax I, McElmurry S, Dossey JE, Miro-Quesada M (1987) Prevention and treatment of sclerosing cholangitis related to chemotherapy delivered by infusaid pump. Proc Am Soc Clin Oncol 6: 89
63. Pariente A, Hamoud A, Goldfain et al. (1989) Hépatites à la clométacine (Dupéran). Etude rétrospective de 30 cas. Un modèle d'hépatite immunoallergique. Gastroenterol Clin Biol 13: 769–774
64. Parry SW, Pelias ME, Browder W (1988) Acalculous hypersensitivity cholecystitis: hypothesis of a new clincopathologic entity. Surgery 104: 911–916
65. Pessayre D, Bichara M, Feldmann G, Degott C, Potet F, Benhamou JP (1979) Perhexiline maleate-induced cirrhosis. Gastroenterology 76: 170–177
66. Pessayre D, Larrey D (1988) Acute and chronic drug-induced hepatitis. Baillere's Clin Gastroenterol 2: 385–422
67. Pessayre D, Larrey D (1988) Mechanisms of drug-induced hepatitis. In: Liver Cells and Drugs. Ed. Guillouzo A, Libbey J London 164: 129–142
68. Pessayre D, Larrey D, Funck-Bretano D, Benhamou JP (1985) Drug interactions and hepatitis produced by some macrolide antibiotics. J Antimicrob Chemother 16 (suppl A): 181–194

69. Pitre J, Houssin D, Louvel A, Vigouroux C, Gaudric M, Chapuis Y (1991) Cho-langite ectasiante et cirrhose biliaire secondaire après chimiothérapie intra-artérielle hépatique. Gastroenterol Clin Biol 15: 350–354
70. Poucell S, Ireton J, Valencia-Mayoral P, Downar E, Larratt L, Patterson J, Blen-dis L, Phillips J (1984) Amiodarone-associated phospholipidosis and fibrosis of the liver. Light, immunohistochemical, and electron microscopic studies. Gastro-enterology 86: 926–936
71. Prescott LF (1983) Paracetamol overdosage. Pharmacological considerations and clinical management. Drugs 25: 290–314
72. Prigrau C, Pahissa A, Gropper S, Sureda D, Martínez-Vásquez JM (1989) Ceftriaxone-associated biliary pseudolithiasis in adults. Lancet 1: 165
73. Review by an International Group (1983) Histopathology of the intrahepatic bili-ary tract. Liver 3: 161–175
74. Rooks JB, Ory HW, Ishak KG, Strauss LT, Greenspan JR, Hill AP, Tyler CW (1979) The cooperative liver tumor study group – epidemiology of hepatocellular adenoma. The role of oral contraceptive use. JAMA 242: 645–648
75. Rougier P (1986) Chimiothérapie intra-artérielle hépatique des métastases iso-lées des adénocarcinomes colo-rectaux. Gastroenterol Clin Biol 10: 122–130
76. Schaad UB, Wedgwood-Krucko J, Tschaeppeler H (1988) Reversible ceftriaxone-associated biliary pseudolithiasis in children. Lancet 2: 1411–1413
77. Seeff LB, Cuccherini BA, Zimmerman HJ, Adler EA, Benjamin SB (1986) Ace-taminophen hepatotoxicity in alcoholics. A therapeutic misadventure. Ann Intern Med 104: 399–404
78. Shear NH, Spielberg SP, Grant DM, Tang BK, Kalow W (1986) Differences in metabolism of sulfonamides predisposing to idiosyncratic toxicity. Ann Intern Med 105: 179–183
79. Simon JB, Manley PN, Brien JF, Armstrong PW (1984) Amiodarone hepatotoxi-city simulating alcoholic liver disease. N Engl J Med 311: 167–172
80. Spes CH, Angermann CE, Beyer RW, Schreiner J, Lehnert P (1990) Increased incidence of cholelithiasis in heart transplant recipients receiving cyclosporin the-rapy. Transplantation 9: 404–407
81. Spielberg SP, Gordon GB, Blake DA, Goldstein DA, Herlong HF (1981) Predis-position to phenytoin hepatotoxicity assessed in vitro. N Engl J Med 305: 722–727
82. Steiner A, Weisser B, Vetter WA (1991) A comparative review of the adverse effects of treatments for hyperlipidaemia. Drug Saftety 6: 118–130
83. Stolzer B, Miller G, White WA, Zuckerbrod M (1950) Postarsenical obstructive jaundice complicated by xanthomatosis and diabetes mellitus. Am J Med 9: 124–132
84. Stricker BHCH, Block R, Claas FHJ, Parys GEV, Desmet VJ (1988) Hepatic injury associated with the use of nitrofurans: a clinicopathological study of 52 reported cases. Hepatology 8: 599–606
85. Stricker BHCH, Spoelstra P (1985) Drug-induced hepatic injury. A comprehen-sive survey of the literature on adverse drug reactions up to January 1985; Else-vier, Amsterdam 1985
86. Valla D, Benhamou JP (1988) Liver diseases related to oral contraceptives. Dig Dis 6: 76–86
87. Valla D, Benhamou JP (1988) Drug-induced vascular and sinusoidal lesions of the liver. Baillere's Clin Gastroenterol 2: 481–500
88. Yeung E, Jackson J, Finn JP, Thomas MG, Benjamin IS, Adam A (1990) Acal-culous cholecystis complicating hepatic intraarterial Lipiodol: case report. Cardi-ovasc Intervent Radiol 12: 80–82
89. Zafrani ES, Pinaudeau Y, Dhumeaux D (1983) Drug-induced vascular lesions of the liver. Arch Intern Med 143: 495–802

90. Zimmerman HJ (1978) Hepatotoxicity. The adverse effects of drugs and other chemicals on the liver. Appleton-Century-Crofts, New York 1978
91. Zimmerman HJ, Lewis JH (1987) Drug-induced cholestasis. Med Toxicol 2: 112–160

Drug-Induced Pancreatitis

C. B. KÖLBEL[1] and M. V. SINGER

Abteilung für Gastroenterologie, Medizinische Klinik, Universitätsklinikum Essen, BRD

1 Introduction

Since 1959, when the first report on drug-induced pancreatitis was published by Johnston and Cornish [58], at least 50 different drugs have been implicated as possible but rare causes of pancreatitis. A convincing causal relationship has been established for only a small number of these drugs while the pathogenesis of this type of pancreatitis remains almost completely elusive. This chapter gives an overview on different aspects of drug-induced pancreatitis. As generally accepted, three categories of drugs are discussed inasfar as their causal relationship with the development of pancreatitis is definite, probable, or possible [73].

The exocrine and the endocrine pancreas has been found to contain cytosolic and microsomal enzymes, among them P450-catalyzed function oxidases and NADPH reductase [110] enabling the pancreas, as the liver, to metabolize different drugs, however, at a lower capacity than the liver [65]. While there is certain information regarding the mechanisms of pancreatic toxicity of chemicals such as alloxan, ethionine, and nitrosamine, most of which has been obtained from studies in rodents, little is known on how drugs induce pancreatitis [110]. The information that we have on drug-induced pancreatitis relies for the most part on clinical reports and occasionally on surveys while animal studies are only occasionally available. Thus a causal relationship is difficult to establish since many patients are treated with several drugs, and for ethical reasons rechallenge studies have rarely been performed. The real incidence of this sometimes fatal complication remains unknown. It is generally assumed that drug-induced pancreatitis is an acute form of pancreatitis, although this has not yet been proven [116].

2 Drug-Induced Pancreatitis: Definite Associations

A drug can be considered definitely to cause pancreatitis if clinical symptoms together with specific laboratory findings occur during treatment with the drug, resolve after its withdrawal, and recur after the patient is rechallenged with the drug. This must be clearly documented. So far only ten drugs fulfill these conditions; these are the following:

Azathioprine
Chlorothiazide
Furosemide
6-Mercaptopurine
Methyldopa
Estrogens
Sulfonamides
Sulindac
Tetracycline
Valproic acid

2.1 Azathioprine

In an analysis of data obtained from the National Cooperative Crohn's Disease Study, Sturdevant et al. [121] have convincingly demonstrated that azathioprine can induce acute pancreatitis. Six out of 113 patients (5.3 %) treated only with azathioprine developed this complication. Several cases have been reported earlier [61, 86, 92]. Reports of pancreatitis in patients who were treated with azathioprine after organ transplantation have also been published. However, these patients were under multiple drug treatment [41]. Frick et al. [43] did not find an association between azathioprine therapy and pancreatitis in their analysis of data prospectively obtained from renal transplantation patients receiving azathioprine and cyclosporine. Pancreatitis has also been reported in patients who received the drug for reasons other than inflammatory bowel disease or transplantation [48]. Pancreatitis develops 2–3 weeks after azathioprine has been started. It is usually mild, and clinical signs of the disease resolve within 10 days after withdrawal of the drug. Rechallenge studies have been performed; patients who stopped taking the drug reported worsening of the symptoms within hours after they had restarted taking it [121]. The mechanisms of azathioprine pancreatitis are unknown. There is probably no dose-response relationship. The latency of symptoms as well as the shortening of the latency period after resuming therapy suggests an allergic mechanism [110, 121].

2.2 Chlorothiazide, Hydrochlorothiazide

Considering the frequency of chlorothiazide prescription, acute pancreatitis is an extremely rare complication of these drugs. It was first reported in 1959 [58] and less than 30 cases have been published so far (for review see [74]). Two cases of pancreatitis have been reported in patients treated with metolazone, a thiazide-like quinazoline diuretic [3, 44]. There is evidence from epidemiological studies that patients with pancreatitis have a higher use of diuretics than controls [12, 80]. Symptoms began 2 weeks – 5 years after the onset of therapy, and pancreatitis was often severe, with several fatalities. Rechallenge studies have been performed in some patients [34]. Seven percent of 300 mice treated with chlorothiazide for up to 6 months developed pancreatitis [27]. There have been speculations that thiazide-induced pancreatitis might be mediated by a mechanism involving calcium metabolism since in some patients suffering from pancreatitis, hypercalcemia, parathyroid hyperplasia, and adenomas have been found [110]. Whether this reflects a real association is doubtful since patients with hyperparathyroidism do not bear a higher risk for pancreatitis than a general hospital population [9].

2.3 Furosemide

Several cases of pancreatitis associated with furosemide therapy have been reported [15, 19, 60, 118, 120, 134], including some with recurrence of pancreatitis after patients had been rechallenged with the drug [19, 60]. Pancreatitis is mostly mild, and symptoms develop after 1 month of therapy. The mechanism by which furosemide causes pancreatitis is unclear. Furosemide has been shown to stimulate potently pancreatic secretion in healthy volunteers [125]. Another mechanism discussed is ischemia due to increased blood viscosity [54].

2.4 6-Mercaptopurine

The active metabolic product of azathioprine is 6-mercaptopurine. The first report of pancreatitis associated with 6-mercaptopurine therapy was published by Heuser et al. in 1967 [51]. Two cases including pancreatitis after the drug had been reintroduced were reported by Bank and Wright [8]. Most cases stem from a study including a total number of 400 patients with inflammatory bowel disease [49, 98]. The authors found that pancreatitis was the most frequent short-term complication of mercaptopurine therapy, occurring in 13 of 400 patients (3.3 %). Pancreatitis was usually mild and occurred in all but one case within 1–5 weeks. Patients rechallenged with the drug developed pancreatitis after a shorter latency than at the initial attack, indicating an allergic mechanism as assumed for azathioprine.

2.5 Methyldopa

Only four patients who developed pancreatitis associated with the treatment of methyldopa have been reported, and were women [104, 128, 131]. Symptoms were mild, and pancreatitis recurred after rechallenge with the drug [74].

2.6 Estrogens

Bank and Marks [8] were the first to describe pancreatitis associated with estrogen therapy. There is now no doubt that there is a definite association between estrogen therapy and pancreatitis regardless the indication for its use. As with other drugs, the incidence of this rare complication remains unclear, and epidemiological studies are not available. In most cases pancreatitis occurred within 3 months after the onset of therapy and was always associated with excessive levels of hypertriglyceridemia [29, 42, 45]. This indicates that most patients had an underlying hyperlipoproteinemia, and that pancreatitis was mediated by hypertriglyceridemia induced by estrogens. Positive rechallenge studies have been reported [29].

2.7 Sulfonamides

Sulfonamides either alone or in combination with other drugs such as sulfamethoxazole trimethoprim [1] or in compound drugs such as sulfa-salazine (salazosulfapyridine) have been found to induce pancreatitis [11, 28, 39, 122]. Positive rechallenge tests have also been reported [4, 73]. In the case reported by Alberti-Flor et al. [1] hemorrhagic pancrea-titis occurred together with fulminant hepatitis. Latency periods lasted 1–2 weeks. As with most other drugs, an allergic mechanism appears to be involved in the development of pancreatitis. This is substantiated by the observation of a patient with sulfonamide-induced pancreatitis in whom lymphocytes were stimulated in vitro by sulfamethoxazole, sulfa-pyridine, and sulfasalazine whereas this stimulation was not observed in a control [13]. Recent observations suggest that some cases of pancreati-tis attributed to the sulfonamide moiety in patients under treatment with salazosulfapyridine may have been induced by 5-aminosalicylic acid.

2.8 Sulindac

Several cases of pancreatitis associated with the therapy of sulindac, a nonsteroidal anti-inflammatory drug, have been published [46, 64, 71, 77, 114]. In addition, about 100 cases of pancreatitis associated with this drug have been reported to the producer [139]. Positive rechallenge tests have been documented in several patients [139]. Pancreatitis, usually mild, develops within the first 5 months of therapy. Only in one case did it occur 5 years after the onset of treatment, indicating that long-term therapy does not exclude this complication [139].

2.9 Tetracycline

Only four cases of tetracycline-induced pancreatitis without evidence of liver abnormalities have been reported [37, 85, 126]. In one of these cases pancreatitis developed at two separate occasions after tetracycline therapy [37]. All four patients had received tetracycline at oral doses of 1–2 g/day. Symptoms usually developed within the first 2 months of ther-apy. Pancreatitis was usually moderate. In most published cases pan-creatitis occurred in association with fatty liver degeneration and renal failure induced by high doses of intravenous tetracycline. Most but not all of these complications were observed in pregnant women treated in the 1950s and 1960s [66, 89, 112]. The mortality rate for mothers was found to be 17 % [66]. The mechanisms by which tetracycline induces pancreatitis are unclear, and speculations on the involvement of a toxic metabolite of this drug must be validated [85].

2.10 Valproic Acid

According to a recently published review [62], 24 patients have been reported who developed pancreatitis attributed to the treatment of valproic acid, most of them children. No dose relationship for the development of this complication has been found, which occurred after a latency period ranging from 2 days to 4.5 years [74]. Two fatal cases of pancreatitis have been published. Several patients had positive rechallenge tests.

3 Drug-Induced Pancreatitis: Probable Associations

A probable causal relationship between drug treatment and the development of pancreatitis is assumed if one of the conditions to prove a causal relationship is not fulfilled. This could, for instance, be a lacking rechallenge test. From the information available different authors might draw different conclusions regarding a causal relationship. The list of drugs for which a probable association with pancreatitis can be said to exist includes the following:

5-Aminosalicylic acid
L-Asparaginase
Chlorthalidone [59]
Cimetidine
Cisplatin
Corticosteroids
Cyclosporine
Cytosine arabinoside
Diphenoxylate [76]
Ethacrynic acid [111]
Hypercalcemia
Methandienone
Metronidazole
Nitrofurantoin [83]
Pentamidine
Polychemotherapy for cancer
Phenformin
Piroxicam [74]
Procainamide [73]

3.1 5-Aminosalicylic Acid

Several cases of pancreatitis have been reported in patients treated with 5-aminosalicylic acid [30, 33, 41, 47, 55, 103, 106]. Positive rechallenge tests have been performed. Pancreatitis has also been observed in patients treated with disodium azodisalicylate [78, 97]. Pancreatitis usually developed after 1–4 weeks of therapy and was clinically mild. Symptoms resolved with discontinuation of therapy. Since symptoms in rechallenge studies recurred after a shorter latency period, an allergic mechanism appears to be involved in the development of pancreatitis [33]. These observations suggest that pancreatitis attributed to the sulfonamide moiety in patients under salazosulfapyridine treatment might have been induced by 5-aminosalicylic acid. The cases described suggest a causal relationship between 5-aminosalicylic therapy and the onset of pancreatitis.

3.2 L-Asparaginase

A high rate of pancreatitis has been associated with L-asparaginase. In nine of ten studies published, pancreatitis was mentioned as a possible and severe complication of this therapy [73]. The complication rate has been reported to range from 8% to 25% [84] and the mortality rate from 1.8% to 4.6% [108]. Different rates of pancreatitis have been reported depending on the type of L-asparaginase used [35]. In most cases pancreatitis occurred while patients were being treated [84], but delayed onsets have been reported [132]. In spite of the high incidence of pancreatitis a convincing proof of a causal relationship is still lacking; no challenge tests have been performed. And patients treated with L-asparaginase usually received a multidrug treatment for serious underlying diseases.

3.3 Cimetidine

In addition to evidence obtained from studies performed in rats [57], three case reports including four patients suggest an association between the development of pancreatitis and the treatment with cimetidine [5, 88, 133]. In spite of the few cases reported the positive challenge test performed in two patients suggests a causal relationship.

3.4 Cisplatin

Only three cases of mild pancreatitis have been reported in association with cisplatin therapy [17, 20, 119]. In addition, Vermorken and Pinedo

[129] reported four cases of hyperamylasemia without clinical symptoms. Rechallenge studies have not been performed.

3.5 Corticosteroids

Since the first report of steroid-induced pancreatitis in 1955 [137] about 50 cases have been published (for review see [117]). Latency periods ranged from 5 days to 7 years of treatment, and fatal outcomes have been reported. One case described in detail developed pancreatitis after rechallenge with the drug [70]. In addition, pancreatitis observed in children under corticosteroid therapy [6, 91, 101] favors the role of this drug as an etiological factor of pancreatitis since this disease is extremely rare among children. An autopsy study performed in patients who received glucocorticoids or ACTH shortly before their deaths showed acute pancreatitis in 29 % [21]. In spite of the numerous reports and the newer positive rechallenge observation a causal relationship has not generally been accepted [117]. First, numerous patients were under additional drug treatment which might have also induced pancreatitis. Second, many patients had serious underlying diseases.

3.6 Cyclosporine

There have been several reports of acute pancreatitis observed in transplantation patients treated with cyclosporine and glucocorticosteroids for immunosuppression [23, 72, 100]. In a follow-up study performed in 466 patients with renal allografts two patients developed acute pancreatitis, three pancreatic abscess, and one pancreatic pseudocyst. Among the patients 5 % developed asymptomatic hyperamylasemia [72], an observation confirmed by Prevost et al. [77]. In a similar study performed in cardiac transplant patients treated with cyclosporine and glucocorticosteroids, 16 out of 86 patients developed acute pancreatitis; two patients died [23]. So far, a convincing causal relationship between cyclosporine treatment and the development of pancreatitis has not been established. Elevated amylasemia and lipasemia observed in patients treated with cyclosporine does not necessarily reflect pancreatitis since both enzymes depend on glomerular filtration rate, which is often impaired in those patients [99]. On the other hand, autopsy studies show elevated concentrations of cyclosporine in the pancreas [102]. Together with a complication rate of 5 % a causal relationship is probable, in spite of the fact that these patients were under concomitant medication.

3.7 Cytosine Arabinoside

Siemers et al. [115] observed two cases of pancreatitis among 30 patients treated with high doses of cytosine arabinoside (10.5–13.8 g/day). Another case of pancreatitis occurred in a young patient while on therapy with a conventional dose of this drug (160 mg/day). Pancreatitis recurred when the patient was rechallenged with the drug [2].

3.8 Iatrogenic Hypercalcemia

Pancreatitis attributed to iatrogenic hypercalcemia has been reported in patients under calcium infusions [53], vitamin D therapy [69], hemodialysis [38], and parenteral nutrition [56]. Fatal cases have not been reported. The cases reported suggest but do not prove pancreatitis since rechallenge tests were not performed.

3.9 Metronidazole

Four cases of pancreatitis have been published related to metronidazole use [26, 95, 109]; three of these occurred in women treated for vaginitis, a fourth for rectovaginal fistula associated with Crohn's disease. A causal relationship has been suspected since pancreatitis recurred upon rechallenge.

3.10 Pentamidine

Numerous patients have been reported who developed pancreatitis associated with pentamidine therapy [63, 81, 90, 93, 107, 130, 135]. Most of them were AIDS patients treated for *Pneumocystis carinii* pneumonia. Pancreatitis usually developed after 1–2 weeks of treatment, often associated with impairment of renal functions and dysglycemia. Recurrence of pancreatitis has been documented after a patient had been rechallenged with the drug. Because of multidrug therapy and the serious underlying disease a causal relationship is hard to prove. In a retrospective case-control analysis performed in children with AIDS, pentamidine therapy was significantly associated with pancreatitis [79]. The mechanism of pentamidine-associated pancreatitis is unknown. However, the development of pancreatitis appears to be dose related since several cases have been reported in France where the daily dose is higher than in the United States. Since pentamidine as a highly lipophilic substance can accumulate in the pancreas [32], discontinuing therapy does not instantly prevent progression of pancreatitis.

3.11 Phenformin

Several cases of phenformin-associated pancreatitis have been reported in the 1970s (for review see [73]). A causal relationship has not been established. So far, no other cases have been published.

3.12 Polychemotherapy for Cancer

Pancreatitis has been observed in patients on cancer polychemotherapy. In addition to the cases reported under single drug treatment, a few patients have been described who developed pancreatitis while on combined therapy with cyclophoshamide, 5-fluorouracil, mitomycin, and methotrexate. Other combinations included cyclophoshamide, vincristine, and doxorubicin. A causal association could not be verified from these observations [74].

4 Drug-Induced Pancreatitis: Possible Associations

A possible association between drug treatment and the development of pancreatitis characterizes reports with inadequate information. In a number of cases patients who developed pancreatitis attributed to a specific drug had concomitant drug treatment, often serious underlying diseases or other causes of pancreatitis had not convincingly been excluded. Such drugs include:

Amoxapine [74]
μ-Blockers (see [74])
Bumetanide [118]
Carbamazepine
Colchizine
Danazol [22]
2',3'-Dideoxyinosine (didanosine)
Erythromycin [124]
Fibrates [113]
Gold [36]
Ibuprofen (see [74])
Interleukin-2
Lipid emulsions
Lovostatin [96]
Mefenamic acid (see [74])
Paracetamol (acetaminophen; see [74])
Phenolphtalein (see [74])
Ranitidine
Salicylates

Ticarcillin/clavulanic acid (see [74])
Cholestyramine, cyproheptadine, diazoxide, histamine, indomethacin, rifampicin, warfarin (see [73, 74])

4.1 Carbamazepine

A few cases of pancreatitis have been attributed to the treatment with this drug. According to Mallory and Kern [74], these cases suggest but do not confirm a causal relationship.

4.2 Colchicine

Two cases of pancreatitis have been attributed to colchicine, but a causal association has not been established (for review see [74]).

4.3 2', 3'-Dideoxyinosine (Didanosine)

2', 3'-Dideoxyinosine is still an experimental antiviral drug for the treatment of AIDS patients. Nevertheless more than 25000 AIDS patients have been treated "on demand" with this drug in the United States [52]. Several reports on dideoxyinosine-related pancreatitis have been published [24, 25, 31, 67, 105, 127]. Pancreatitis has been reported in 2.5 % of 19000 patients treated with moderate doses (5–10 mg/kg per day) of this drug [14]. In a retrospective analysis of a prospective clinical trial including 51 patients with AIDS treated with high doses (10–12 mg/kg per day) pancreatitis was observed in 24 % ; in addition, asymptomatic elevation of pancreatic enzymes was found in 39 % of the patients. Challenge tests performed in two of the patients yielded positive results. However, all patients who developed pancreatitis were on pentamidine and acyclovir treatment [75]. Others have reported pancreatitis in 8.5 % of the patients [136] or up to 47 % when patients received daily doses of up to 66 mg [67]. Pancreatitis occurred within the first 6 months of treatment and was sometimes fatal. The mechanism of dideoxyinosine-associated pancreatitis is unclear, although it appears to be dose related. A causal relationship is suspected, but since most of the seriously ill patients were under additional drug therapy further confirmation must be awaited.

4.4 Interleukin-2

Birchfield et al. [10] reported two cases of acute pancreatitis attributed to interleukin-2 immunotherapy in patients with malignant melanoma.

Both patients received concomitant medications including indomethacin, acetaminophen, and ranitidine, and one of them furosemide. The authors mentioned five other patients who developed an asymptomatic elevation of serum lipase or amylase. One of those patients did not develop any signs of pancreatitis upon rechallenge. These observations do not prove a causal relationship; further reports should be awaited.

4.5 Lipid Infusions

Several cases of pancreatitis have been attributed to lipid infusions [16, 87]. In one case, well-documented pancreatitis recurred upon rechallenge [68]. Further reports should be awaited before a causal association can be established.

4.6 Ranitidine

One case of pancreatitis associated with ranitidine has been described [50]. Two further episodes of pancreatitis recurred upon rechallenge with the drug. A second case of ranitidine-associated pancreatitis has been documented but not published [50]. Further observations must confirm these reports before a causal relationship can be established.

4.7 Salicylates

Three cases of pancreatitis associated with salicylate poisoning have been published]18, 123], and a causal relationship has been suggested [74].

References

1. Alberti-Flor JJ, Hernández ME, Ferrer JP, Howell S, Jeffers L (1989) Fulminant liver failure and pancreatitis associated with the use of sulfamethoxazole-trimethoprim. Am J Gastroenterol 84: 1577–1579
2. Altman AJ, Dinndorf P, Quinn JJ (1982) Acute pancreatitis in association with cytosine arabinoside therapy. Cancer 49: 1386
3. Anderson PE, Ellis GG Jr, Austin SM (1991) Case report: metolazone-associated hypercalcemia and acute pancreatitis. Am J Med Sci 302: 235–237
4. Antonow DR (1986) Acute pancreatitis associated with trimethoprim-sulfamethoxazole. Ann Intern Med 104: 363–365
5. Arnold F, Doule PJ, Bell G (1978) Acute pancreatitis in a patient treated with cimetidine. Lancet i: 382–383
6. Baar HS, Wolff OH (1957) Pancreatic necrosis in cortisone-treated children. Lancet 1: 812–815

7. Bank S, Marks IN (1970) Hyperlipaemic pancreatitis and the pill. Postgrad Med J 46: 576–588

8. Bank L, Wright JP (1984) 6-Mercaptopurine-related pancreatitis in 2 patients with inflammatory bowel disease. Dig Dis Sci 29: 357–359

9. Bess MA, Edis AJ, van Heerden JA (1980) Hyperparathyroidism and pancreatitis: chance or a causal association? JAMA 243: 246–247

10. Birchfield GR, Ward JH, Redman BG, Flaherty L, Samlowski WE (1990) Acute pancreatitis associated with high-dose interleukin-2 immunotherapy for malignant melanoma. West J Med 152: 714–716

11. Block MB, Genant HK, Kirsner JB (1970) Pancreatitis as an adverse reaction to salicylazosulfapyridine. N Engl J Med 282: 380–382

12. Bourke JB, Langman MJS (1980) Do diuretics cause pancreatitis? [letter] Gastroenterology 79: 774

13. Brazer SR, Medoff JR (1988) Sulfonamide-induced pancreatitis. Pancreas 3: 583–586

14. Bristol-Myers Squibb Pharmaceutical Research Institute (1991) ddI-Quarterly Safety Summary.

15. Buchanan N, Cane RD (1977) Furosemide-induced pancreatitis. Br Med J 2: 1417

16. Buckspan R, Woltering E, Waterhouse G (1984) Pancreatitis induced by intravenous infusion of a fat emulsion in an alcoholic patient. South Med J 77: 251–252

17. Bunin N, Meyer WH, Christensen M, Pratt CB (1985) Pancreatitis following cisplatin: a case report [letter]. Cancer Treat Rep 69: 236–237

18. Cabooter M, Elewaut A, Barbier F (1981) Salicylate-induced pancreatitis. Gastroenterology 80: 214–215

19. Call T, Malarkey WB, Thomas FB (1977) Acute pancreatitis secondary to furosemide with associated hyperlipidemia. Am J Dig Dis 22: 835–838

20. Calvo DB, Patt YZ, Wallace S, Chuang VP, Benjamin RS, Pritchard JD, Hersh EM, Bodey GP, Mavligit GM (1980) Phase I-II trial of percutaneous intra-arterial cis-diammine dichloroplatinum (II) for regionally confined malignancy. Cancer 45: 1278–1238

21. Carone F, Liebon A (1957) Acute pancreatic lesion in patients treated with A.C.T.H. and adrenal corticoids. N Engl J Med 257: 690–697

22. Chevalier X, Awada H, Baetz A, Amor B (1990) Danazol induced pancreatitis and hepatitis. Clin Rheumatol 9: 239–241

23. Colon R, Frazier OH, Kahan BD, Radovancevic B, Duncan JM, Lorber MI, Van Buren CT (1988) Complications in cardiac transplant patients requiring general surgery. Sugery 103: 32–38

24. Connolly KJ, Allan JD, Fitch H, Jackson-Pope L, McLaren C, Canetta R, Groopman JE (1991) Phase I study of 2', 3'-dideoxyinosine administered orally twice daily to patients with AIDS or AIDS-related complex and hematologic intolerance to zidovudine. Am J Med 91: 471–478

25. Cooley TP, Kunches LM, Saunders CA, Ritter JK, Perkins CJ, McLaren C, McCaffrey RP, Liebman HA (1990) Once-daily administration of 2', 3'-dideoxyinosine (ddI) in patients with the acquired immunodeficiency syndrome or AIDS-related complex. Results of a phase I trial. N Engl J Med 322: 1340–1345

26. Corey WA, Doebbeling BN, DeJong KJ, Britigan BE (1991) Metronidazole-induced acute pancreatitis. Rev Infect Dis 13: 1213–1215

27. Cornish AL, McClellan JT, Johnston DH (1961) Effects of chlorothiazide on the pancreas. N Engl J Med 265: 673–675

28. Das KM, Eastwood MA, McManus JP, Sircus W (1973) Adverse reactions during salicylazosulfapyridine therapy and the relation with drug metabolism and acetylator phenotype. N Engl J Med 289: 491–495

29. Davidhoff F, Tishler S, Rosoff C (1973) Marked hyperlipemia and pancreatitis associated with oral contraceptive therapy. N Engl J Med 289: 552–555

30. Deprez P, Descamps C, Fiasse R (1989) Pancreatitis induced by 5-aminosalicylic acid [letter]. Lancet 2 (8660): 445–446
31. Dolin R, Lambert JS, Morse GD, Reichman RC, Plank CS, Reid J, Knupp C, McLaren C, Pettinelli C (1990) 2', 3'-Dideoxyinosine in patients with AIDS or AIDS-related complex. Rev Infect Dis 12 (Suppl 5): S 540–549
32. Donnelly H, Bernard EM, Rothkotter H, Gold JWM, Armstrong D (1988) Distribution of pentamidine in patients with AIDS. J Infect Dis 157: 985–989
33. Eckardt VF, Kanzler G, Rieder H, Ewe K (1991) 5-Aminosalicylsäure-assoziierte Pankreatitis. Dtsch Med Wochensch 116: 540–542
34. Eckhauser ML, Dokler M, Imbembo AL (1987) Diuretic-associated pancreatitis: a collective review and illustrative cases. Am J Gastroenterol 82: 865–870
35. Eden OB, Shaw MP, Lilleyman JS, Richards S (1990) Non-randomised study comparing toxicity of Escherichia coli and Erwinia asparaginase in children with leukaemia. Med Pediatr Oncol 18: 497–502
36. Eisemann AD, Becker NJ, Miner PB Jr, Fleming J (1989) Pancreatitis and gold treatment of rheumatoid arthritis [letter]. Ann Intern Med 111: 860–861
37. Elmore M, Rogge J (1981) Tetracycline-induced pancreatitis. Gastroenterology 81: 1134–1136
38. Evans DB, Slapak M (1975) Pancreatitis in the hard water syndrome. Br Med J 3: 748
39. Faintuch J, Mott CB, Machado MC (1985) Pancreatitis and pancreatic necrosis during sulfasalazine therapy. Int Surg 70: 271–272
40. Fernández JA, Rosenberg JC (1976) Post-transplantation pancreatitis. Surg Gynecol Obstet 143: 795–798
41. Fiorentini MT, Fracchia M, Galatola G, Barlotta A, de la Pierre M (1990) Acute pancreatitis during oral 5-aminosalicylic acid therapy. Dig Dis Sci 35: 1180–1182
42. Foster ME, Powell DEB (1975) Pancreatitis, multiple infarcts and oral contraception. Postgrad Med J 51: 667–669
43. Frick TW, Fryd DS, Goodale RL, Simmons RL, Sutherland DE, Najarian JS (1991) Lack of association between azathioprine and acute pancreatitis in renal transplantation patients [letter]. Lancet 337: 251–252
44. Fuchs JE Jr, Keith MR, Galanos AN (1989) Probable metolazone-induced pancreatitis [letter]. DICP 23: 711
45. Glueck CJ, Scheel D, Fishback J, Steiner P (1972) Estrogen-induced pancreatitis in patients with previously covert familialtype V hyperlipoproteinemia. Metabolism 21: 657–666
46. Goldstein J, Laskin DA, Ginsberg GH (1980) Sulindac associated with pancreatitis (letter). Ann Intern Med 93: 151
47. Grimaud JC, Maillot A, Bremondy A, Thervet L, Salducci J (1989) Faut-il toujours accuser la sulfapyridine? A propos d'un cas de pancréatite aiguë induite par la mésalazine. Gastroent Clin Biol 13: 432
48. Guillaume P, Grandjean E, Male PJ (1984) Azathioprine-associated acute pancreatitis in the course of chronic active hepatitis. Dig Dis Sci 29: 78–79
49. Haber CJ, Meltzer SJ, Present DH, Korelitz BI (1986) Nature and course of pancreatitis caused by 6-mercaptopurine in the treatment of inflammatory bowel disease. Gastroenterology 91: 982–986
50. Herrmann R, Shaw RG, Fone DJ (1990) Ranitidine-associated recurrent acute pancreatitis. Aust N Z J Med 20: 243–244
51. Heuser E, Lieberman E, Donnell GN, Landing BH (1967) Subcutaneous fat necrosis with acute hemorrhagic pancreatitis: a case in a child with steroid-resistant nephrosis treated with 6-mercaptopurine. California Med 106: 58–63
52. Hirschel B, Vanhems P (1991) Anti-retrovirale Therapie in der Schweiz 1991. Schw Med Wschr 121: 1187–1193
53. Hochgelerent EL, Davis DS (1974) Acute pancreatitis secondary to calcium infusion in a dialysis patient. Arch Surg 108: 218–219

54. Holland SD, Williamson HE (1984) Acute effects of high-ceiling diuretics on pancreatic blood flow and function. J Pharmacol Exp Ther 229: 440–446
55. Isaacs KL, Murphy D (1990) Pancreatitis after rectal administration of 5-aminosalicylic acid. J Clin Gastroenterol 12: 198–199
56. Izsak ME, Shike M, Roulet M, Jeejeebhoy KN (1980) Pancreatitis in association with hypercalcemia in patients receiving total parenteral nutrition. Gastroenterology 79: 555–558
57. Joffe S, Lee FK (1978) Acute pancreatitis after cimetidine administration in experimental duodenal ulcers. Lancet 1: 383
58. Johnston DH, Cornish AL (1959) Acute pancreatitis in patients receiving chlorothiazide. JAMA 170: 2054–2056
59. Jones MF, Caldwell JR (1962) Acute hemorrhagic pancreatitis associated with the administration of chlorthalidone. N Engl J Med 267: 1029–1031
60. Jones PE, Oelbaum MH (1975) Furosemide-induced pancreatitis. Br Med J 1: 133–134
61. Kawanishi H, Rudolph E, Bull FE (1973) Azathioprine-induced acute pancreatitis. N Engl J Med 289: 357
62. Kayemba Kay's Kabangu S, Bovier Lapierre M, Jalaguier E (1991) Acute pancreatitis and valproic acid. Pédiatrie 46: 839–843 (in French)
63. Klatt EC (1992) Pathology of pentamidine-induced pancreatitis. Arch Pathol Lab Med 116: 162–164
64. Klein SM, Khan MA (1983) Hepatitis, toxic epidermal necrolysis and pancreatitis in association with sulindac therapy. J Rheumatol 10: 512–513
65. Kokkinakis DM, Scarpelli DG, Rao MS, Hollenberg PF (1983) Metabolism of the pancreatic carcinogens N-nitroso-2,6-dimethylmorpholine and N-nitrosobis(2-oxopropyl)amine by microsomes and cytosol of hamster pancreas and liver. Cancer Res 43: 5761–5767
66. Kunelis CT, Peters JL, Edmondson HA (1965) Fatty liver of pregnancy and its relationship to tetracycline therapy. Am J Med 38: 359–377
67. Lambert JS, Seidlin M, Reichman RC, Plank CS, Laverty M, Morse GD, Knupp C, McLaren C, Pettinelli C, Valentine FT, Dolin R (1990) 2', 3'-Dideoxyinosine (ddI) in patients with the acquired immunodeficiency syndrome or AIDS-related complex. A phase I trial. N Engl J Med 322: 1333–1340
68. Lashner BA, Kirsner JB, Hanauer SB (1986) Acute pancreatitis associated with high-concentration lipid emulsion during total parenteral nutrition therapy for Crohn's disease. Gastroenterology 90: 1039–1041
69. Leeson PM, Fourman P (1966) Acute pancreatitis from vitamin D poisoning in a patient with parathyroid deficiency. Lancet 1: 1185–1186
70. Levine RA, McGuire RF (1988) Corticosteroid-induced pancreatitis: a case report demonstrating recurrence with rechallenge. Am J Gastroenterol 83: 1161–1164
71. Lilly EL (1981) Pancreatitis after administration of sulindac (letter). JAMA 246: 2680
72. Lorber MI, Van Buren CT, Flechner SM, Williams C, Kahan BD (1987) Hepatobiliary and pancreatic complications of cyclosporine therapy in 466 renal transplant recipients. Transplantation 43: 35–40
73. Mallory A, Kern F (1980) Drug-induced pancreatitis: a critical review. Gastroenterology 78: 813–820
74. Mallory A, Kern F (1980) Drug-induced pancreatitis. Baillieres Clin Gastroenterol 2: 293–307
75. Maxson CJ, Greenfield SM, Turner JL (1992) Acute pancreatitis as a common complication of 2', 3'-dideoxyinosine therapy in the acquired immunodeficiency syndrome. Am J Gastroenterol 87: 708–713
76. McCormick PA, O'Donoghue D, Brennan N (1985) Diphenoxylate and pancreatitis [letter]. Lancet 1 (8431): 752
77. Memon AN (1982) Pancreatitis and sulindac (letter). Ann Intern Med 97: 139

184   C. B. Kölbel and M. V. Singer

78. Meyers S (1988) Disodium azodisalicylate and sulfasalazine [letter]. Am J Gastroenterol 83: 1187
79. Miller TL, Winter HS, Luginbuhl LM, Orav EJ, McIntosh K (1992) Pancreatitis in pediatric human immunodeficiency virus infection. J Pediatr 120: 223–227
80. Moir DC (1978) Drug-associated acute pancreatitis. Lancet ii: 369–370
81. Murphey SA, Josephs AS (1981) Acute pancreatitis associated with pentamidine therapy. Arch Intern Med 141: 56–58
82. Murphy RL, Noskin GA, Ehrenpreis ED (1990) Acute pancreatitis associated with aerosolized pentamidine. Am J Med 88: 53N–56N
83. Nelis GF (1983) Nitrofurantoin-induced pancreatitis: report of a case. Gastroenterology 84: 1032–1034
84. Nguyen DL, Wilson DA, Engelman ED, Sexauer CL, Nitschke R (1987) Serial sonograms to detect pancreatitis in children receiving L-asparaginase. South Med J 80: 1133–1136
85. Nicolau DP, Mengedoht DE, Kline JJ (1991) Tetracycline-induced pancreatitis. Am J Gastroenterol 86: 1669–1671
86. Nogueira JR, Freedman MA (1972) Acute pancreatitis as a complication of Imuran therapy in regional enteritis. Gastroenterology 62: 1040–1041
87. Noseworthy J, Colodny AH, Eraklis AJ (1983) Pancreatitis and intravenous fat: an association in patients with inflammatory bowel disease. J Ped Surg 18: 269–272
88. Nott DM, de Sousa BA (1989) Suspected cimetidine-induced acute pancreatitis. Br J Clin Parct 43: 264–265
89. Ober WB, LeCompte PM (1955) Acute fatty metamorphosis of the liver associated with pregnancy. Am J Med 19: 743–758
90. O'Neil MG, Selub SE, Hak LJ (1991) Pancreatitis during pentamidine therapy in patients with AIDS. Clin Pharm 10: 56–59
91. Oppenheimer EH, Boitnott JK (1960) Pancreatitis in children following adrenal corticosteroid therapy. Bull Johns Hosp 107: 297–306
92. Paloyan D, Levin B, Simonowitz D (1977) Azathioprine-associated acute pancreatitis. Am J Dig Dis 22: 839–840
93. Pauwels A, Eliaszewicz M, Larrey D, Lacassin F, Poirier JM, Meyohas MC, Frottier J (1990) Pentamidine-induced acute pancreatitis in a patient with AIDS. J Clin Gastroenterol 12: 457–459
94. Picon M, Causse X, Gelas P, Retornaz G, Trepo C, Bouletreau P (1991) Hépatite aiguë sévère à la pentamidine au cours du traitement d'une pneumocystose liée au SIDA (letter). Gastroenterol Clin Biol 15: 463–464
95. Plotnick BH, Cohen I, Tsang T, Cullinane T (1985) Metronidazole-induced pancreatitis. Ann Intern Med 103: 891–892
96. Pluhar W (1989) Ein Fall möglicher Lovostatin-induzierter Pankreatitis bei gleichzeitigem Gilbert-Syndrom. Wien Klin Wchschr 101: 551–554
97. Poldermans D, van Blankenstein M (1988) Pancreatitis induced by disodium azodisalicylate. Am J Gastroenterol 83: 578–580
98. Present DH, Meltzer SJ, Krumholz MP, Wolke A, Korelitz BI (1989) 6-Mercaptopurine in the management of inflammatory bowel disease: short- and long-term toxicity. Ann Intern Med 111: 641–649
99. Prevost X, Myara I, Cosson C, Duboust A, Moatti N (1988) Asymptomatic hyperamylasemia after cyclosporine therapy in patients with renal transplants. Transplant Proc 20: 555–558
100. Przepiorka D, Shapiro S, Schwinghammer TL, Bloom EJ, Rosenfeld CS, Shadduck RK, Venkataramanan R (1991) Cyclosporine and methylprednisolone after allogeneic marrow transplantation: association between low cyclosprine concentration and risk of acute graft-versus-host disease. Bone Marrow Transplant 7: 461–465
101. Reimenschneider TA, Wilson JF, Vernier RL (1968) Glucocorticoid-induced pancreatitis in children. Pediatrics 41: 428–437

102. Ried M, Gibbons S, Kwok D et al. (1983) Cyclosporine levels in human tissues of patients treated for one week to one year. Transplant Proc 15 (suppl 1): 2434
103. Romero Castro R, Jiménez Saenz M, Pellicer Bautista FJ, Domínguez Palomo S, Herrerias Gutiérrez JM (1991) Pancreatitis acuda por acido 5-aminosalicilico. Rev Esp Enferm Dig 79: 219–221
104. Rominger JM, Gutiérrez JG, Curtis D, Chey WY (1978) Methyldopa-induced pancreatitis. Am J Dig Dis 23: 756–758
105. Rozencweig M, McLaren C, Beltangady M, Ritter J, Canetta R, Schacter L, Kelley S, Nicaise C, Smaldone L, Dunkle L et al. (1990) Overview of phase I trials of 2', 3'-dideoxyinosine (ddI) conducted on adult patients. Rev Infect Dis 12 (Suppl 5) S570–S575
106. Sachedina B, Saibil F, Cohen LB, Whittey J (1989) Acute pancreatitis due to 5-aminosalicylate. Ann Intern Med 110: 490–492
107. Salmeron S, Petitpretz P, Katlama C, Herve P, Brivet F, Simonneau G, Duroux P, Regnier B (1986) Pentamidine and pancreatitis [letter]. Ann Intern Med 105: 140–141
108. Samuels BI, Culbert SJ, Okamura J et al. (1976) Early detection of chemotherapy-related pancreatic enlargement in children using abdominal sonography. A preliminary report. Cancer 38: 1515–1523
109. Sanford KA, Mayle JE, Dean HA, Greenbaum DS (1988) Metronidazole-associated pancreatitis. Ann Intern Med 109: 756–757
110. Scarpelli DG (1989) Toxicology of the pancreas. Toxicol Appl Pharmacol 101: 543–554
111. Schmidt P, Friedman IS (1967) Adverse effects of ethacrynic acid. NY State J Med 67: 1438–1442
112. Schultz JC, Adamson JS, Workman WW, Norman TD (1963) Fatal liver disease after intravenous administration of tetracyline in high dosage. N Engl J Med 269: 999–1004
113. Sgro C, Escousse A (1991) Side effects of fibrates (except liver and muscle). Thérapie 46: 351–354 (in French)
114. Siefkin AD (1980) Sulindac and pancreatitis (letter). Ann Intern Med 93: 932–933
115. Siemers RF, Friedenberg WR, Norfleet RG (1985) High-dose cytosine arabinoside-associated pancreatitis. Cancer 56: 1940–1942
116. Steer ML (1989) Classification and pathogenesis of pancreatitis. Surg Clin North Am 69: 467–480
117. Steinberg WM, Lewis JH (1981) Steroid-induced pancreatitis: Does it really exist? Gastroenterology 81: 799–808
118. Stenvinkel P, Alvestand A (1988) Loop diuretic-induced pancreatitis with rechallenge in a patient with malignant hypertension and renal insufficiency. Acta Med Scand 224: 89–91
119. Stewart DJ, Feun LG, Maor M, Leavens M, Burgess MA, Benjamin RS, Bodey GP Sr (1983) Weekly cisplatin during cranial irradiation for malignant melanoma metastatic to brain. J Neurooncol 1: 49–51
120. Strunge P (1975) Furosemide-induced pancreatitis? Br Med J 1: 434
121. Sturdevant RAL, Singleton JW, Deren JJ, Law DH, McCleery JL (1979) Azathioprine-related pancreatitis in patients with Crohn's disease. Gastroenterology 77: 883–886
122. Suryapranata H, DeVries H (1986) Pancreatitis associated with sulphasalazine. Br Med J 292: 732
123. Sussman S (1963) Severe salicylism and acute pancreatitis. Calif Med 99: 29–32
124. Teillet L, Chaussade S, Mory B, Roche H, Couturier D, Guerre J (1991) Pancréatite aiguë associée a une antibiothérapie par l'erythromycine intraveneuse (letter). Gastroenterol Clin Biol 15: 265–266
125. Thomas FB, Falko JM, Caldwell JH, Mekhjian HS (1975) Effects of furosemide on pancreatic exocrine function. Gastroenterology 68: 998

126. Torosis J, Vender R (1987) Tetracycline-induced pancreatitis. J Clin Gastroenterol 9: 580–581
127. Valentine FT, Seidlin M, Hochster H, Laverty M (1990) Phase I study of 2', 3'-dideoxyinosine: experience with 19 patients at New York University Medical Center. Rev Infect Dis 12 (Suppl 5): S534–539
128. Van der Heide H, ten Haaft MA (1981) Pancreatitis caused by methyldopa. Br Med J 282: 1930–1931
129. Vermorken JB, Pinedo HM (1982) Gastrointestinal toxicity of cis-diammine dichloroplatinum. II. Personal observations. Neth J Med 25: 270–274
130. Villamil A, Hammer RA, Rodríguez FH (1991) Edematous pancreatitis associated with intravenous pentamidine. South Med J 84: 796–798
131. Warren SE, Mitas JA, Swerdlin AHR (1980) Pancreatitis due to methyldopa: case report. Military Med 145: 399–400
132. Weetman RM, Baehner RL (1974) Latent onset of clinical pancreatitis in children receiving L-asparaginase therapy. Cancer 34: 780–785
133. Wilkinson ML, O'Driscoll R, Kiernan TJ (1981) Cimetidine and pancreatitis. Lancet i: 610–611
134. Wilson AE, Mehra SK, Gomersall CR (1967) Acute pancreatitis associated with furosemide therapy. Lancet 1: 1355
135. Wood G, Wetzig N, Hogan P, Whitby M (1991) Survival from pentamidine induced pancreatitis and diabetes mellitus. Aust N Z J Med 21: 341–342
136. Yarchoan R, Pluda JM, Thomas RV, Mitsuya H, Brouwers P, Wyvill KM, Hartman N, Johns DG, Broder S (1990) Long-term toxicity/activity profile of 2', 3'-dideoxyinosine in AIDS or AIDS-related complex. Lancet 336: 526–529
137. Zion MM, Goldberg B, Suzman MM (1955) Corticotrophin and cortisone in the treatment of scleroderma. Q J Med 24: 215–217
138. Zuger A, Wolf BZ, el-Sadr W, Simberkoff MS, Rahal JJ (1986) Pentamidine-associated fatal acute pancreatitis. JAMA 256: 2383–2385
139. Zygmunt DJ, Williams HJ, Bienz SR (1986) Acute pancreatitis associated with long-term sulindac therapy. West J Med 144: 461–462

Gastrointestinal Damage by Cancer Chemotherapy

M. VALENTINI, R. CANNIZZARO, F. BORTOLUZZI, M. SOZZI,
M. FORNASARIG, and E. BERTOLISSI

Division of Gastroenterology and Digestive Endoscopy, Regional Cancer Center,
Aviano, Italy

Injury to the gastrointestinal tract may occur with any number of chemotherapy drugs used for the treatment of malignant disease. Indeed, the dosage of antineoplastic drugs is limited by toxic effects not only on the lungs, kidneys, and bone marrow but also on the liver and gastrointestinal tract. Some gastrointestinal symptoms such nausea, vomiting, anorexia, abdominal pain, and diarrhea may be either the presenting features of the underlying malignancy, usually self-limiting adverse reactions to drugs, or in some cases manifestations of more severe chemotherapy-induced gastrointestinal toxicity. Anticancer drugs as a group are thought preferentially to attack rapidly dividing tissues, including the gastrointestinal mucosa: nevertheless, remarkable little attention has been directed to the gastrointestinal epithelium and to its function in man.

1 Nausea and Vomiting

Nausea and vomiting are the more common gastrointestinal side effects induced by chemotherapy and may represent a significant obstacle to the optimal care of cancer patients. As Penta et al. [56] and Laszlo [39] have pointed out, 10 %–30 % of patients refuse chemotherapy because of nausea and vomiting and an additional 20 % delay treatment or miss clinical appointments because of fear of emesis. Chemotherapy-related nausea and vomiting play an important role in patients with cancer for the following reasons:

- They can lead to discontinuation of chemotherapy unless controlled [40].
- They are dose-limiting toxic effects for a great number of antineoplastic agents [36].
- They may promote other complications such as anorexia, dehydratation, metabolic imbalance, and psychological depression [21, 31, 51].
- Their control is an essential aspect of patient compliance with chemotherapic treatment [32].
- They are significant elements in the evaluation of the results of clinical trials of chemotherapic drugs [54]. Several factors affect the frequency and severity of emesis: age, sex, alcohol intake, motion sickness, emetic response to prior chemotherapy, and type and dose of antineoplastic drug used [42, 52].

Younger patients seem to have increased anticipatory nausea and vomiting and an increased incidence of dystonic reactions [37]. Women are more often affected by nausea and vomiting than men [60]. Susceptibility to motion sickness and poor previous emetic control may increase nausea and vomiting. Emesis seems to be more easily controlled in patients with a history of heavy chronic alcohol intake [14, 76].

1.1 Pathophysiology of Emesis

The vomiting response is coordinated and controlled by the "vomiting center," located in the medullary reticular formation posterior to the fourth ventricle [6]. This center receives impulses from the gastrointestinal tract, liver, pharynx, cerebral cortex, and chemoreceptor trigger zone (CTZ), located in the area postrema, adjacent to the vomiting center.

Three mechanisms have been postulated [70] for activating the CTZ: a) a direct action of the emetogenic agent to cells in the area postrema, b) an indirect action via afferent nerves entering the area postrema, and c) an indirect action via humoral factors released as a result of chemotherapy. The main pathway from the gut to the central nervous system is via the vagus nerve [26]. Chemotherapeutic drugs or their metabolites may be detected by the CTZ and may release 5-

hydroxytryptamine (5-HT) from the gastrointestinal tract which may depolarize vagal nerve afferents [1]. Many different types of receptors, such as those for acetylcholine, dopamine, histamine, noradrenaline, adrenaline, and serotonin may be involved in the emetic reflex, and their relative importance depends on different aetiologies of emesis [1].

Recently, some reports have demonstrated the importance of the 5-HT_3 receptor in the control of chemotherapy- and radiotherapy-induced emesis, with important therapeutic consequences [43, 58, 64, 78].

1.2 Clinical Findings

The time of onset of emesis after chemotherapy administration varies. Acute nausea and vomiting occur during the first 24 h following chemotherapy and are related to the chemotherapic agent used, its emetogenicity, the prior experience, and the antiemetic regimens [26, 42]. For example, cisplatin induces nausea and vomiting after 1–6 h, whereas high-dose cyclophosphamide after 6–12 h [24]. Delayed emesis, which is normally less severe, occurs 24 h–7 days after the start of treatment [37, 42, 61]. Some patients who experience chemotherapy-induced emesis may have anticipatory nausea and vomiting before undergoing subsequent courses of treatment [27]. This probably conditioned reaction may also be triggered by chemotherapy-associated odors, tastes, or thoughts [26].

1.3 Emetic Potential

The severity and frequency of emesis are related to the emetic potential and to the dose of the chemotherapic agent used. A recent hypothesis suggests that the emetogenic potential is related to the ability of the drugs to damage DNA; therefore the compounds that do not damage DNA (e. g., vinca alkaloids, antiestrogens) have a low emetogenic potential.

A classification system of the emetogenic potential of single chemotherapeutic agents, also related to drug dosages, has been proposed by Lindley et al. [42]. Antineoplastic drugs have been classified into five groups, with high (>90 %), moderately high (60 %–90 %), moderate (30 %–60 %), moderately low (10 %–30 %), and low (<10 %) emetogenicity. Table 1 contains a simplified classification of the emetic potential of the more common chemotherapy drugs.

In the combination antineoplastic therapies the frequency and severity of emesis is usually similar to that induced by the drug with the highest emetic potential.

Table 1. Emetogenic potential of the most used chemotherapy drugs

Emetogenic potential	Antineoplastic drugs	
High	Cisplatin	Pentostatin
	Dacarbazine	Streptozocin
	Cyclophosphamide (>1 g)	Doxorubicin
	Cytarabine	Mitomycin
	Carmustine	Procarbazine
	Lomustine	Daunorubicin
	Meclorethamine	Actinomycin D
Moderate	Doxorubicin	5-Azacytidine
	Methotrexate	Asparaginase
	Cyclophosphamide (<1 g)	Bleomycin
	5-Fluorouracil	Hydroxyurea
	Vinblastine	Etoposide
Low	Vincristine	Chlorambucil
	Busulfan	Tamoxifen
	Thioguanine (oral)	Cyclophosphamide (oral)

1.4 Therapy of Emesis

As noted above, patients who suffered from incomplete acute control of nausea and vomiting at their first cycle of chemotherapy are more likely to develop delayed emesis [37, 42, 61] or anticipatory emesis at subsequent cycles [27, 50]. Therefore, antiemetic treatment should be directed toward complete prevention of the first emetic episode at the start of chemotherapy treatment.

A variety of antiemetic drugs have been used to treat chemotherapy-induced emesis:

1.4.1 Phenothiazines

These agents are basically apomorphine inhibitors and therefore presumably have their mode of action in blocking the action of the CTZ. Some derivatives (e. g., chlorpromazine) may also act by depression of the vomiting center. Phenothiazines are used for moderate to mild emesis and are usually well tolerated. However, the control of nausea and vomiting is often unsatisfactory.

1.4.2 Butyrophenones

These drugs are also thought to act by the blockade of the CTZ. Haloperidol and droperidol are the most useful of butyrophenones in controlling vomiting and nausea and seem to be more effective than phenothia zines. These agents are generally well tolerated, with a low incidence of side effects such as sedation and hypotension and relatively higher incidence of extrapyramidal reactions when given in higher doses.

1.4.3 Corticosteroids

The mechanism of action of these agents (dexamethasone, methylprednisolone) in controlling emesis is poorly understood; it seems to be related to the inhibition of prostanoid synthesis. Nevertheless they have well-defined antiemetic activity, more relevant in combination with other antiemetic medications (phenothiazines, butyrophenones, metoclopramide, 5-HT$_3$ receptor antagonists) than as single agents. Side effects are usually mild and well tolerated.

1.4.4 Benzodiazepines

The agent most carefully studied to date is lorazepam. It does not appear to have direct antiemetic activity, but through its anxiolytic and amnesic properties it can be an important factor for the patient's comfort in decreasing anticipatory nausea and eliminating the memory of unpleasant emetic episodes. Not all benzodiazepines are equally able to treat chemotherapy-induced emesis. Kearsley et al. [35] reported in a perspective, randomized, crossover study with lorazepam, oxazepam, and methylprednisolone in patients taking cisplatin chemotherapy that those receiving lorazepam had fewer episodes of severe vomiting and preferred this regimen to the two others.

1.4.5 Cannabinoids

These drugs seem to have a role in managing chemotherapy-induced emesis among young patients with a history of drug use. Among older patients cannabinoids (tetraidrocannabinol and nabilone) are not well tolerated because of side effects such as loss of control and altered sensation.

1.4.6 Substitute Benzamides

Metoclopramide is the most commonly used agent in this class. It has significant efficacy in preventing and controlling both moderate and severe chemotherapy-induced emesis. Metoclopramide is thought to act primarily by dopaminergic receptor blockade (and, as recently suggested, by serotonin receptor blockade) as well as stimulation of gastroduodenal motility and gastric emptying. The most common side effects are diarrhea, sedation, and, particularly if high dosages are used, extra-pyramidal reactions. Several recent studies have assessed the efficacy of high-dose metoclopramide in cisplatin-induced emesis, whether administered as continuous infusion [15, 53, 80] or by mouth.

1.4.7 5-HT₃ Receptor Antagonists

Development of the new class of antiemetic agents, the 5-HT$_3$ receptor antagonists, represents an important advance in the management of nausea and vomiting associated with moderately to severely emetogenic chemotherapy regimes. The most studied 5-HT$_3$ receptor antagonists are ondasentron and granisetron, but other compounds are under development. In several trials ondasentron as single agent was demonstrated to be superior to metoclopramide in terms of efficacy, toxicity, and patient compliance for the prevention of nausea and vomiting in two-thirds to three-quarters of patients receiving cisplatin regimens [22, 45, 55, 71]. Cunningham et al. [13] and Smith et al. [72] performed non randomized clinical trials in which the combination of dexamethasone and ondasentron seemed to potentiate the latter's antiemetic efficacy. Granisetron is a highly selective and potent 5-HT$_3$ antagonist developed for the management of emesis. It has been shown to prevent nausea and vomiting in approximately 60 % of patients receiving high-dose cisplatin [75] and in approximately 75 % of patients treated with moderately emetogenic cytostatic chemotherapy [72].

Several studies [7, 9, 16, 45, 46] compared the efficacy and safety of granisetron as single agent with combinations of conventional antiemetic therapies (metoclopramide plus dexametasone, chlorpromazine plus dexametasone, alizapride plus dexametasone) in patients receiving high or moderate emetogenic chemotherapy or fractionated chemotherapy. In these studies the percentage of complete responders was higher or significantly higher in the granisetron group. Headache was the most frequently reported adverse event. Due to the lack of published studies directly comparing the efficacy of granisetron and ondasentron, Dilly [17] compared the two compounds by a review of the literature, suggesting a 15 % difference in the control of cisplatin-induced emesis and a 30 % difference in the control of fractionated chemotherapy-induced emesis in favor of granisetron.

2 Esophageal and Gastroduodenal Injury

Enhancement of radiation injury to the esophagus has been reported [49] with a number of chemotherapeutic agents, including actinomycin D, doxorubicin, carmustine, bleomycin, 5-fluorouracil, hydroxyurea, procarbazine, and vinblastine. More severe reactions have been observed when chemotherapy and radiation therapy are performed concomitantly.

Severe esophagitis resulting in stricture may occur following concomitant doxorubicin and radiation therapy for lung cancer [4, 8, 29]. In the series of Bereton et al. [8] 28 of 50 patients with small cell carcinoma of the lung, treated with irradiation and concurrent combination chemotherapy containing doxorubicin developed moderate to severe (in three with esophageal stricture) esophagitis.

A "recall phenomenon" [18, 19] has been described in patients receiving actinomycin D and doxorubicin following irradiation; recurrent esophagitis and stricture developed weeks to months after radiation therapy.

Chemotherapeutic agents affect rapidly proliferating cells and may produce mucositis at any level in the upper gastrointestinal tract. Mucositis is usually caused by methotrexate, antibiotics, 5-fluorouracil, and vinca alkaloids. The toxicity of methotrexate seems to depend on the duration of exposure to the drug more than on peak levels [3]. Hepatic arterial infusion of 5-fluorouracil with surgical implanted pumps may cause severe dyspepsia with erosive gastritis, gastric and duodenal ulcers, and duodenitis in 10%–50% of patients [2, 68], perhaps also depending on the different surgical techniques [33]. In fact, an important role seems to be related to the chemical arteriolitis associated with inadvertent infusion of the drug in the gastric and duodenal arteries [47].

Hemorragic gastritis with upper gastrointestinal bleeding is rarely a complication of chemotherapy. The risk of bleeding appears to be inversely related to platelet count [10]. Gastritis may also be caused by exogenous irritants such as steroids, but bleeding usually stops with discontinuation of the drugs [67].

3 Small-Bowel Toxic Reactions

Chemotherapy agents may cause injury to the small intestine by a variety of mechanisms, including morphologic and functional abnormalities of intestinal absorptive cells, malabsorption, and intramural hematomas of the small bowel. Trier [77] studied the ultrastructural alterations involving mithocondria, endoplasmic reticulum, and Golgi apparatus in small-intestinal epithelium in patients receiving a single dose of methotrexate intravenously. These changes were not associated with absorptive abnormalities. Changes in the ultrastructure of the small bowel have been found in patients who received single doses of methotrexate by mouth [30] and combination chemotherapy with methotrexate, cyclophosphamide, and 5-fluorouracil, without consistent absorptive abnormalities [66].

Slavin et al. [69] described a clinical syndrome that included abdominal pain, diarrhea, ileus, melena, or hematochezia and protein-losing enteropathy in a group of 33 patients 8–11 days after starting treatment with cytosine arabinoside (ara-C) in combination with a variety of other agents.

Vascular changes such as teleangiectasias, intramural hematomas, and extensive mucosal necrosis have been associated with regimens including ara-C. These vascular changes may persist for several weeks and may predispose to intestinal infections by fungi and bacteria, leading to pneumatosis cystoides intestinalis, sepsis, peritonitis, and liver abscess. No similar mucosal alterations were reported in other studies with combination chemotherapies that do not include ara-C [66, 74].

Despite the previously discussed structural changes in the small-bowel mucosa caused by chemotherapy, symptoms are often transient.

Watery or bloody diarrhea may occur with numerous antineoplastic drugs, such as 5-florourouracil, methotrexate, hydroxyurea, nitrosourea, and alkylating agents, particularly after high-dose regimens.

Malabsorption is an uncommon side effect of chemotherapy. Malabsorption subsequent to inhibition of intestinal mucosal cell renewal leading to blunting of intestinal villi [23] and decreased D-xylose absorption [11] have been documented during methotrexate therapy, but normal absorptive function of the small intestine has been described in patients receiving various chemotherapy regimens [74]. McDonald and Tirumali [48] suggested that the ability of the small bowel to absorb nutrients may be related to rapid repair of damage and to the large functional reserve of the small intestine.

4 Colonic Injury

Three types of necrotizing colitis have been described by Dosik et al. [20]: pseudomembranous colitis, ischemic necrosis and agranulocytic colitis. Pseudomembranous colitis due to *Clostridium difficile* toxin [12] or to other toxin-producing organisms [25, 57] has been described in patients receiving antineoplastic drugs. However, since the concomitant administration of antibiotics is common in these patients, colitis might be related both to antibiotic treatment and to chemotherapy drugs. The etiology of the ischemic necrosis, found at autopsy in patients who received combination chemotherapy, is probably multifactorial.

Agranulocytic colitis (typhlitis), which involves the cecum and right colon in patients with severe neutropenia [59] has been described by Wagner et al. [79] in children receiving chemotherapy for leukemia.

Constipation in patients receiving chemotherapy may be related to diminished oral intake or to concomitant opiates or anticholinergic medication [48]. Constipation, abdominal pain, and adynamic ileus are reported [34, 62, 63, 81] as neurotoxic side effects of vinca alkaloids. The neurotoxic syndrome is more frequent and severe in patients treated with the highest dose [34]; elderly patients are more predisposed to these toxicities. A high mortality rate has been reported in patients with colonic pseudoobstruction [65]. Symptoms may appear within 3 days of vincristine administration and usually resolve, if treated conservatively, over several weeks. Mild laxatives and stool softeners may represent the prophylactic treatment of constipation.

5 Conclusions

Chemotherapy-induced gastrointestinal side effects represent a significant problem for patients with cancer. Nausea and vomiting are surely the most frequent symptoms; they depend primarily on the action of the drugs on the central nervous system rather than directly on the gastrointestinal mucosa.

High dosages of prokinetic agents may exert a good symptomatic effect in low and moderate emesis, and the new 5-HT$_3$ antagonists seem to represent a major advance in the management of highly ematogenetic chemotherapies.

Chemotherapic agents may also cause mucosal injury to the whole gastrointestinal tract. Related symptoms are typical and often transient but must be taken into account when starting a chemotherapeutic regimen in cancer patients.

References

1. Andrews PLR, Rapeport WG, Sanger GJ (1988) Neuropharmacology of emesis induced by anti-cancer therapy. Trends in Pharmacol Sci 9: 334–341
2. Ansfield FJ, Ramírez G (1978) The clinical results of 5-fluorouracil intrahepatic arterial infusion in 528 patients with metastatic cancer to the liver. Prog Clin Cancer 7: 201–206
3. Bleyer WA (1978) The clinical pharmacology of methotrexate. Cancer 41: 36–51
4. Blum RH, Carter SK (1974) Adriamycin: a new anticancer drug with significant clinical activity. Ann Int Med 80: 249–259
5. Borison HL, McCarthy LE (1983) Neuropharmacology of chemotherapy induced emesis. Drugs 2 (Suppl 1): 8–17
6. Borison HL, Wang WC (1953) Physiology and pharmacology of vomiting. Pharmacol Rev 5: 193–230
7. Bremer K on behalf of the Granisetron Study Group (1992) A single-blind comparative study with alizapride plus dexamethasone in the prophylaxis and control of emesis in patients receiving cytostatic therapy over a 5-day treatment period. Eur J Cancer 28: 1018–1022
8. Brereton HD, Kent CH, Johnson RE (1979) Chemotherapy and radiation therapy for small cell cancer of the lung: a remedy for past therapeutic failure. In: Muggia F, Rozencweig M (eds) Lung cancer: progress in therapeutic research. Raven, New York

9. Chevallier B, on behalf of the Granisetron Study Group (1990) Efficacy and safety of granisetron compared with high-dose metoclopramide plus dexamethasone in patients receiving high-dose cisplatin in a single-blind study. Eur J Cancer 26 (Suppl 1): S 33–S 37
10. Chu DZJ, Shivshanker K, Stoehlien JR et al. (1983) Thrombocytopenia and gastrointestinal hemorrhage in the cancer patient: prevalance of unmarked lesions. Gastrointest Endosc 29: 269–272
11. Craft AW, Kay HZM, Lawson DN et al. (1977) Methotrexate-induced malabsorption in children with acute lymphoblastic leukemia. BMJ 2: 1511–1512
12. Cudmore MA, Silva J, Fekety R et al. (1982) Clostridium difficile colitis associates with cancer chemotherapy. Arch Intern Med 142: 333–335
13. Cunningham D, Turner A, Hawthorn et al. (1989) Ondasentron with and without dexamethasone to treat chemotherapy-induced emesis (editorial), Lancet i: 1323
14. D'Acquisto RW, Tyson LB, Gralla RJ et al. (1986) The influence of a chronic high alcohol intake on chemotherapy-induced nausea and vomiting. Proc Am Soc Clin Oncol 5: 257
15. Dana BW, McDermott M, Everts E et al. (1987) A randomized trial of high dose bolus metoclopramide versus low-dose continuous infusion metoclopramide in the prevention of cisplatin induced emesis. Am J Clin Oncol 10: 253–256
16. Diehl V on behalf of the Granisetron Study Group (1992) Fractionated chemotherapy-granisetron or conventional antiemetics?. Eur J Cancer 28 A (Suppl 1): S 21–S 28
17. Dilly S (1992) Are granisetron and ondasentron equivalent in the clinic? Eur J Cancer 28 A (Suppl 1): S 32–S 35
18. Donaldson SS, Glick JM, Wilbur SR (1974) Adriamycin activating a recall phenomenon after radiation therapy. Ann Intern Med 81: 407–408
19. Donaldson SS, Lenon RA (1979) Alteration of nutritional status: the impact of chemotherapy and radiation therapy. Cancer 43: 2036–2052
20. Dosik GM, Luna M, Valdivieso M et al. (1979) Necrotizing colitis in patients with cancer. Am J Med 67: 646–656
21. Durant JR (1984) The problem of nausea and vomiting in modern cancer chemotherapy. CA 34: 2–6
22. Einhorn LE, Nagy C, Werner K et al. (1990) Ondasentron: a new antiemetic for patients receiving cisplatin chemotherapy. J Clin Oncol 8: 731–735
23. Faloon WW (1970) Drug production of intestinal malabsorption. NY State J Med 70: 2189–2192
24. Fetting JH, Grochow LB, Folstein MF et al. (1982) The course of nausea and vomiting after high dose cyclophosphamide. Cancer Treat Rev 66: 1487–1493
25. Freeman HJ, Rabeneck L, Owen D (1981) Survival after necrotizing enterocolitis of leukemia treated with oral vancomycin. Gastroenterology 81: 791–794
26. Freeman AJ, Cullen MH (1991) Advances in the management of cytotoxic drug-induced nausea and vomiting. J Clin Pharm Ther 16: 411–421
27. Gralla RJ, Tyson LB, Kriss MG et al. (1987) The management of chemotherapy induced nausea and vomiting. Med Clin North Am 71: 289–301
28. Gralla RJ (1989) An outline of anti-emetic treatment. Eur J Cancer 25 (Suppl 1): S 7–S 11
29. Greco FA, Brereton HD, Kent H et al. (1976) Adriamycin and enhanced radiation reaction in normal esophagus and skin. Ann Intern Med 85: 294–298
30. Gwavava NJT, Pinkerton CR, Glasgow JFT et al. (1981) Small bowel enterocyte abnormalities caused by methotrexate treatment in acute lymphoblastic leukemia of childhood. J Clin Pathol 34: 790–795
31. Harris JG (1978) Nausea, vomiting and cancer treatment. CA 28: 194–201
32. Hoagland AC, Morrow GR, Bennet JM et al. (1983) Oncologists views of cancer patient noncompliance. Am J Clin Oncol 6: 239–244

33. Hohn DC, Stagg RJ, Price DC et al. (1985) Avoidance of gastroduodenal toxicity in patients receiving hepatic arterial 5-fluoro-2'-deoxyuridine. J Clin Oncol 3 (N. 9): 1257–1260
34. Holland JF, Scharlau C, Gailani S et al. (1973) Vincristine treatment of advanced cancer: a cooperative study of 392 cases. Can Res 33: 1258–1264
35. Kearsley JH, Williams AM, Fiumara AM (1989) Antiemetic superiority of lorazepam over oxazepam and methylprednisolone as premedicants for patients receiving cisplatin-containing chemotherapy. Cancer 64: 1595–1599
36. Krakoff IH (1987) Cancer chemotherapeutic agents. CA 37: 93–105
37. Kris MG, Tyson LB, Gralla RJ (1983) Extrapyramidal reactions with high-dose metoclopramide. N Engl J Med 309: 433
38. Kris MG, Gralla RJ, Clark RA et al. (1985) Incidence, course, and severity of delayed nausea and vomiting following the administration of high-dose cisplatin. J Clin Oncol 3: 1379–1384
39. Laszlo J (ed) (1983) Antiemetics and cancer chemotherapy. Williams and Wilkins, Baltimore, pp. 1–5
40. Laszlo J, Lucas VS (1981) Emesis as a critical problem in chemotherapy. N Engl J Med 305: 148–149
41. Lewis JH et al. (1986) Gastrointestinal Injury Due to Medicinal Agents. Am J Gastroenterol 9: 819–834
42. Lindley CM, Bernard S, Fields SM (1989) Incidence and duration of chemotherapy-induced nausea and vomiting in the outpatient oncology population. J Clin Oncol 7: 1142–1149
43. Marty M (1989) Ondasentron in the prophylaxis of acute cisplatin induced nausea and vomiting. Eur J Cancer 25 (Suppl 1): S 41–S 45
44. Marty M on behalf of the Granisetron Study Group (1990) A comparative study of the use of granisetron, a selective 5HT-3 antagonist, versus a standard antiemetic regimen of chlorpromazine plus dexamethasone in the treatment of cytostatic-induced emesis. Eur J Cancer 26: S 28–S 33
45. Marty M, Pouillart P, Scholl S et al. (1990) Comparison of the 5-hydroxytryptamine 3 (serotonin) antagonist ondasentron (GR 38032F) with high-dose metoclopramide in the control of cisplatin-induced emesis. N Engl J Med 322: 816–821
46. Marty M, On behalf of the Granisetron Study Group (1992) A comparison of granisetron as a single agent with conventional combination antiemetic therapies in the treatment of cytostatic-induced emesis. Eur J Cancer 28 A (Suppl 1): S 12–S 16
47. Mavligit GM, Faintuch J, Levin B et al. (1987) Gastroduodenal mucosal injury during hepatic arterial infusion of chemotherapeutic agents. Gastroenterology 92: 566–569
48. McDonald GB, Tirumali N (1984) Intestinal and liver toxicity of antineoplastic drugs. West J Med 140: 250–259
49. Mitchell EP, Schein PS (1982) Gastrointestinal toxicity of chemotherapeutic agents. Semin Oncol 9: 52–644
50. Morrow GR (1982) Prevalence and correlates of anticipatory nausea and vomiting in chemotherapy patients. J Natl Cancer Inst 68: 585–588
51. Morrow GR (1987) Management of nausea in the cancer patient. In: Rosenthal S, Carignan JR, Smith BD (eds) Medical care of the cancer patient. Saunders, Philadelphia, pp. 381–388
52. Morrow GR (1989) Chemotherapy-Related Nausea and Vomiting: Etiology and Management. CA 39: 102–103
53. Navari RM (1989) Comparison of intermittent versus continuous infusion metoclopramide in control of acute nausea induced by cisplatin chemotherapy. J Clin Oncol 7: 943–946
54. Olver IN, Simon RM, Aisner J (1986) Antiemetic studies: a methodological discussion. Cancer Treat Rep 70: 555–563

198   M. Valentini et al.

55. Pendergrass K, Hainsworth J, Harvey W et al. (1990) Ondasentron (OND): more effective than metoclopramide (MCP) in the prevention of cisplatin (DDP)-induced nausea (N) and vomiting (V). Proc Am Soc Clin Oncol 9: 319
56. Penta J, Poster D, Bruno S (1983) The pharmacologic treatment of nausea and vomiting caused by cancer chemotherapy: a review. In: Laszlo J (ed) Antiemetics and cancer chemotherapy. Williams and Wilkins, Baltimore, pp. 53–92
57. Philips RKS, Glazer G, Borriello SP (1981) Non-Clostridium difficile pseudomembranous colitis responding to both vancomycin and metronidazole. BMJ 283: 823
58. Priostman TJ (1989) Clinical studies with ondasentron in the control of radiation induced emesis. Eur J Cancer 25 (Suppl 1): S 29–S 33
59. Riddell RH (1982) The gastrointestinal tract. In: Riddell RD (ed) Pathology of drug-induced and toxic disease. Churchill Livingstone, New York, pp. 515–605
60. Roila F, Tonato M, Basurto C et al. (1987) Anti-emetic activity of high-doses of metoclopramide alone in cisplatin treated cancer patients: a randomized double-blind trial of the Italian oncology group for clinical research. J Clin Oncol 5: 141–149
61. Roila F, Boschetti E, Tonato M et al. (1991) Predictive factors of delayed emesis in cisplatin-treated patients and antiemetic activity and tolerability of metoclopramide or dexamethasone. Am J Clin Oncol 14: 238–242
62. Rosenthal S, Kaufman S (1975) Vincristine neurotoxocity. Ann Intern Med 80: 733–737
63. Sandler SG, Tobin W, Henderson ES (1969) Vincristine induced neuropathy: a clinical study of fifty leukemia patients. Neurology (Minneapolis) 19: 367–374
64. Schmoll HJ (1989) The role of ondasentron in the treatment of emesis induced by non-cisplatin-containing chemotherapy regimens. Eur J Cancer 25 (Suppl 1): S 35–S 39
65. Schoenfield LF, Lachin JM (1981) The Steering Committee. Chenodiol (chenodeoxycholic acid) for dissolution of gallstones: The National Cooperative Gallstone Study. A controlled trial of efficacy and safety. Ann Intern Med 95: 257–282
66. Shaw MT, Spector MH, Ladman AJ (1979) Effects of cancer, radiotherapy and cytotoxic drugs on intestinal structure and function. Cancer Treat Rev 6: 141–151
67. Sherlock P (ed) (1979) Effect of cancer treatment on nutrition and gastrointestinal function. Clin Bull 9: 136–145
68. Shike M, Gillin JS, Kemeny N et al. (1986) Severe gastroduodenal ulcerations complicating hepatic artery infusion chemotherapy for metastatic colon cancer. Am J Gastroenterol 81: 176–179
69. Slavin RE, Dias MA, Saral R (1979) Cytosine arabinoside induced gastrointestinal toxic alterations in sequential chemotherapeutic protocols. A clinic pathologic study of 33 patients. Cancer 42: 1747–1759
70. Sledge GW (1990) Chemotherapy-induced nausea and vomiting. Curr Opin Oncol 2: 909–914
71. Sledge GW, Einhorn LH, Nagy C et al. (1990) Randomized trial of ondasentron (OND) and metoclopramide (MCP) as antiemetic therapy for cisplatin-based chemotherapy. Proc Am Soc Clin Oncol 9: 323
72. Smith DB, Newlands ES, Spruyt OW et al. (1990) Ondasentron (GR38032F) plus dexamethasone: effective anti-emetic prophylaxis for patients receiving cytotoxic chemotherapy. Br J Cancer 61: 323–324
73. Smith IE on behalf of the Granisetron Study Group (1990) A comparison of two dose levels of granisetron in patients receiving moderately emetogenic cytostatic chemotherapy. Eur J Cancer 26 (Suppl 1): S 20–S 24
74. Smith FP, Kisner DL, Widerlite L et al. (1979) Chemotherapeutic alteration of small intestinal morphology and function: a progress report. J Clin Gastroenterol 1: 203–207

75. Soukop M on behalf of the Granisetron Study Group (1990) Comparison of two dose levels of granisetron in patients receiving high-dose cisplatin. Eur J Cancer 26 (Suppl 1): S 16–S 20
76. Sullivan JR, Leyden MJ, Bell R (1983) Decreased cisplatin-induced nausea and vomiting with chronic alcohol ingestion. N Engl J Med 309: 796
77. Trier JS (1962) Morphologic alterations induced by methotrexate in the mucosa of human proximal intestine. Gastroenterology 43: 407–424
78. Tyers MB, Bunce KT, Humphrey PPA (1989) Pharmacological and anti-emetic properties of ondasentron. Eur J Cancer 25 (Suppl 1): S 15–S 19
79. Wagner ML, Rosenberg HS, Fernbach DJ et al. (1970) Typhlitis: a complication of leukemia in childhood. AJR 109: 341–350
80. Warrington PS, Allan SG, Cornbleet MA et al. (1988) Optimizing anti-emesis in cancer chemotherapy: efficacy of continuous versus intermittent infusion of high dose metoclopramide in emesis induced by cisplatin. BMJ 293: 1334–1337
81. Weiss H, Walker M, Wiernik P (1974) Neurotoxicity of commonly used antineoplastic agents. N Engl J Med 291: 75–81, 127–133

Afterword: Methodological Problems in Detecting the Risk of Drug Reactions

M. J. S. LANGMAN

Department of Medicine, Queen Elizabeth Hospital, Birmingham, U.K.

The various chapters in this book provide an updated overview of the current body of knowledge about the untoward effects of drugs on the digestive system. As the reader has surely noticed, in some instances the available information seems clear enough, and the number of convincing reports is high, but in other cases reports are anecdotal, and the relationship between drug intake and subsequent phenomena remains uncertain. Thus the chances of assessing the risk of pharmacological adverse effects in a clinical setting are scarce unless a more systematic way of reporting and evaluating drug reactions is employed.

Even if we consider such a well-documented and widely accepted example as peptic ulcer induced by a nonsteroidal anti-inflammatory drug (NSAID), a number of methodological problems become evident.

In assessing the chances it is necessary to define what we mean by risk, to examine the features which provide convincing evidence of causality and to determine whether the studies available are of a sufficient standard to be compelling.

1 Definitions of Risk

1.1 Relative Risk

This expresses the increased, or decreased, chances of developing a condition as a multiple of the chances ordinarily prevailing in the community. A figure of 2.0 indicates a doubling and one of 3.0 a tripling, whereas one of 0.5 indicates a halving. This quantum, also known as the odds ratio, does not give the actual risk, nor on its own can it give the burden of disease imposed by the factor under consideration.

These concepts are best illustrated concretely. If in a particular investigation 40 of 200 patients with haematemesis or melaena due to peptic ulceration prove to have taken an NSAID whereas 20 of 180 appropriately matched controls were also exposed, the relative risk or virtually equivalent odds ratio can be calculated as follows: the proportion of *exposed/nonexposed patients* multiplied by the proportion of *nonexposed/exposed controls*. In the present example this would be: (40/160) (160/20) = 2.00. This does not tell us about absolute risk, only the increased multiple of an unknown base.

It is also important to realise that a risk ratio, when elevated, does not necessarily imply a causal relationship to disease occurrence. The risk factor may be associated but not causal. Thus, in studies of relationships between smoking and disease it is necessary to take account of coincident alcohol consumption and to use methods of study which allow their individual quantification as possible risk factors. Even when this is done, it is still necessary to review criteria which might imply causality.

1.2 Actual Risk

To determine this requires knowledge of two factors: a) the underlying chances of disease in the absence of the factor, and b) whether data exist indicating the chances of disease when the factor is operating in addition to any other known risk factor.

Thus, consider a situation in which patients taking a NSAID who are known to have episodes of ulcer bleeding or perforation at a rate of say, one in every 3000 scripts. Data are uninterpretable without knowing the background rate of disease occurrence in matched nontakers. If this in one in 6000, the conclusion of increased risk in takers is clear, provided sample sizes in those studied are adequate to engender confidence, and provided study populations are comparable. In this context it is necessary to remember that population studies are observational and nonrandomized. It therefore behooves the investigator to check that groups are comparable, for instance in age, sex and any possibly important behavioural characteristics.

Convincing data need to meet certain criteria which match those generally applied in seeking causal relationships epidemiologically. These criteria include the consistency of the relationship, its presence in association with a particular lesion or lesions, a temporal association, a dose-response association, the ability to deny alternative explanation by confounding influences, the existence of a plausible mechanistic explanation, and a fall in risk when the factor is removed.

2 Consistency and Association with Particular Lesions

Older data, concerned mainly with aspirin, emphasized the association between drug use and gastric rather than duodenal lesions. These findings seem likely to have arisen in part or even mainly because it was impossible to inspect the duodenum directly. As a consequence, duodenal disease may have been underemphasized, and the term NSAID gastropathy was coined.

Results obtained in the past 5 years emphasise generally that there is an increased risk of gastric and duodenal ulcer or their complications or of death from them. The strength of the relationship, in the order of a doubling to a quintupling, appears roughly the same. If the relative risk appears much the same for complication occurrence and for death, we can deduce that NSAID exposure is unlikely to affect the course of the lesion, only its establishment. Data for duodenal ulcer differ slightly, some apparently indicating that risk of the disease per se is not increased, although the confidence intervals around the relative risk are compatible with a raised risk as for gastric ulcer; however, the risk of complications seems uniformly raised.

Taken overall, the findings cast doubt on the validity of the limited concept of NSAID gastropathy. Comparison with data for aspirin also suggests that both gastric and duodenal risks differ little from those for non-aspirin NSAIDs. Such findings contrast with experimental studies which have consistently indicated that aspirin is more damaging to the mucosa than nonaspirin NSAIDs in short-term experiments, and that gastric damage is particularly easily demonstrable.

3 Temporal Association

Any disease which is drug induced must have a consistent and reasonable temporal association. This might also mean that risk is associated with duration of exposure. However, at least as far as aspirin is concerned, recent exposure seems to be particularly important. Examination epidemiologically is complicated by the associated concept of adaptive cyto-protection. This postulates that exposure generates a nullifying defensive reaction so that longer duration of exposure leads to reduced risk. Clinical evidence to support such a belief is rather limited. Thus it is difficult, for example, when faced with a declining risk with increased duration of exposure, to decide whether this results from a protective response or from the selective removal of a susceptible population (for instance, giving up treatment because of dyspepsia).

Examination of time trends nationally may also be used as a means of examining coincidence between disease occurrence and drug prescription, but it must be remembered that a multiplicity of factors may be operative simultaneously. Coincidence cannot be accepted as necessarily implying causality.

4 Dose Response

In most circumstances, except where idiosyncratic drug reactions are occurring, one might expect a dose-response relationship on the basis that progressively greater interference with a specific mechanism causes disease increasingly frequently.

5 Confounding Influences

It is of prime importance that comparability between exposed and nonexposed individuals be taken into account. Thus the risk of ulcer complications and death increase greatly in the elderly, and risks may differ in men and women. Other possibly important factors, although proof is inadequate, include alcohol consumption, smoking and poor social circumstances.

In examining data it is important to consider these factors as well as simple design flaws. Were similar search methods for drug use employed in cases and controls? Were controls contemporaneous? Was prescribed and nonprescribed drug use taken into account in both groups? Would hospital or community controls be more appropriate?

6 Mechanistic Explanations

Epidemiological studies may be the first clue to an important cause of disease. However, their cogency is weakened if an underlying mechanism is lacking. In the case of NSAIDs this is perhaps the least of the problems; indeed a multiplicity of mechanisms compete for pre-eminence.

7 Protection by Removal of Exposure

Reduction in smoking results in a fall in the death rate from smoking-related diseases. If an influence is important as a major risk factor, its removal is expected to reduce disease burden. Alternatively, specific protective measures may be employed. If these work, they give convincing support to the causal hypothesis.

Taken overall, even data concerning the association between NSAIDs and ulcer disease are not sufficiently satisfactory from a methodological point of view. The situation is totally unsatisfactory when we consider drug-induced side effects on organs such as the mouth, pancreas, etc.

In conclusion, the state-of-the-art understanding of drug-induced damage to the digestive system makes us realise that much work must be done in the future to obtain systematic and complete information by means of a correct methodological approach.

Subject Index

Springer-Verlag
and the Environment

We at Springer-Verlag firmly believe that an international science publisher has a special obligation to the environment, and our corporate policies consistently reflect this conviction.

We also expect our business partners – paper mills, printers, packaging manufacturers, etc. – to commit themselves to using environmentally friendly materials and production processes.

The paper in this book is made from low- or no-chlorine pulp and is acid free, in conformance with international standards for paper permanency.

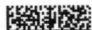